Luminous, playful, intimate, poetic and surprising—this book will touch you, it will take you over, take you inside yourself and outside yourself. It invites you to lose yourself in the material, relational fleshiness of life. Wyatt catches moments of being and becoming in the way only great writers can do. He experiments with thinking otherwise, and asks the reader to encounter the words on the page so they (and you) come alive, escaping into the new, the unexpected, and the vital. He takes you inside a magic circle where anything can happen—and does.

Bronwyn Davies, Emeritus Professor,
Western Sydney University

Jonathan Wyatt's Therapy, Stand-Up, and the Gesture of Writing *comes to me like a compelling poem. In general, the book is about the unfolding and enfolding of therapy, stand-up and writing, and indeed the book teaches me a great deal about those subjects, but it is equally about thinking and feeling in the ongoing process of becoming. It is a poetic gift. Its gentle rhythms find their own form. Its language surrounds, seduces. Its "creative-relational inquiry," to use Wyatt's rich term, opens new ways of moving through the world.*

Ronald J. Pelias, Professor Emeritus,
Southern Illinois University

This is a wonderful book; a book full of elicitations of wonder. Jonathan writes in a style that is seductively conversational, a style that is imbued with affect in a book that never stumbles into proclivities of simply human concerns and emotional response. The book is powerfully energised by the everyday; Jonathan is a hugely adept storyteller and so these vignettes, accounts and exemplifications carry the reader with them into almost unwitting engagements with exciting, profound theorisings with practices of life and facilitations of worlding. Here there are encounters inhabited and animated by clients, family, audiences at stand-up gigs and, through enunciations of these, Jonathan offers diffractive pathways into practices of creative-relational inquiry. This is a book that picks you up, then needs to be carried and can't be put down.

Ken Gale, Lecturer, University of Plymouth, UK

I love this book. It is going to be a classic in our field. The writing is so inviting, so visceral, so open. The topics the book explores are familiar ones, but Wyatt looks at them in fresh ways that are inspiring both to senior researchers and to those new to qualitative inquiry. And I have never read a better introduction to Deleuze and Guattari: he makes their vocabulary understandable at an ethnographic, bodily and emotional level. I especially love Wyatt's metaphors, like the idea of the 'white chalk circle' on the floor for the stand-up comedian being also understood as the chalk circle in a therapeutic session, and in the writer's relationships with real and imagined co-writers and readers. All these are sacred spaces where surprises might happen. One of the things about the book I loved is how Wyatt handles the issue of 'trust'. We trust the therapist, the writer, the stand-up. That trust is necessary for qualitative researchers to do their work, and with trust comes other ethical questions: What do we reveal? What do we hide? How do we decide? I trust that Jonathan has led us towards creative-relational inquiry. That is what is most important.

Laurel Richardson, Professor Emerita, Ohio State University

This book is a wholly original gesture at a world of circuits breathing with the rhythms of something happening, refrains working thresholds of matter and meaning. An ordinary room is a milieu of compositions: the this-ness of the mic, the alcohol, the weather, that shirt. A beautiful, brilliant book, it catches up the reader in the worldly thinking of a shoulder shrugged, a joke, the resonance of a word in a room.

Kathleen Stewart, Professor, University of Texas at Austin

The form and content of Therapy, Stand-up, and the Gesture of Writing offers embodied insight into a creative-relational inquiry revealing new paths in the development of qualitative methodologies. With deft reflexivity Wyatt reveals connections and slippages among seemingly disparate experiences of therapy, humor, and writing as inquiry; such connections are a hallmark of groundbreaking qualitative research. This is a transdisciplinary must-read for writers and researchers.

Tami Spry, Professor, St. Cloud State University

Therapy, Stand-Up, and the Gesture of Writing

Therapy, Stand-Up, and the Gesture of Writing is a sharp, lively exploration of the connections between therapy, stand-up comedy, and writing as a method of inquiry; and of how these connections can be theorized through the author's new concept: *creative-relational inquiry*. Engaging, often poignant, stories combine with rich scholarship to offer the reader provocative, original insights.

Wyatt writes about his work as a therapist with his client, Karl, as they meet and talk together. He tells stories of his experiences attending comedy shows in Edinburgh and of his own occasional performances. He brings alive the everyday profound through vignettes and poems of work, travel, visiting his mother, mourning his late father, and more. The book's drive, however, is in bringing together therapy, stand-up, and writing as a method of inquiry to mobilize theory, drawing in particular from Deleuze and Guattari, the new materialisms, and affect theory. Through this diffractive work, the text formulates and develops *creative-relational inquiry*.

With its combination of fluent story-telling and smart, theoretical propositions, *Therapy, Stand-Up, and the Gesture of Writing* offers compelling possibilities both for qualitative scholars who have an interest in narrative, performative, and embodied scholarship, and those who desire to bring current, complex theories to bear upon their research practices.

Jonathan Wyatt is Professor of Qualitative Inquiry and Director of the Centre for Creative-Relational Inquiry at The University of Edinburgh. Originally an English teacher and youth worker, he worked for ten years as a counsellor in a doctors' surgery alongside being Head of Professional Development at the University of Oxford, before heading north to Scotland in 2013.

Writing Lives
Ethnographic Narratives
Series Editors: Arthur P. Bochner, Carolyn Ellis and
Tony E. Adams
University of South Florida and Northeastern Illinois University

Writing Lives: Ethnographic Narratives publishes narrative representations of qualitative research projects. The series editors seek manuscripts that blur the boundaries between humanities and social sciences. We encourage novel and evocative forms of expressing concrete lived experience, including autoethnographic, literary, poetic, artistic, visual, performative, critical, multi-voiced, conversational, and co-constructed representations. We are interested in ethnographic narratives that depict local stories; employ literary modes of scene setting, dialogue, character development, and unfolding action; and include the author's critical reflections on the research and writing process, such as research ethics, alternative modes of inquiry and representation, reflexivity, and evocative storytelling. Proposals and manuscripts should be directed to *abochner@usf.edu, cellis@usf.edu* or *aeadams3@neiu.edu*.

Other volumes in this series include:

Therapy, Stand-Up, and the Gesture of Writing
Towards Creative-Relational Inquiry
Jonathan Wyatt

Talking White Trash
Mediated Representations and Lived Experiences of White Working-Class People
Tasha R. Dunn

For a full list of titles in this series, please visit: www.routledge.com/Writing-Lives-Ethnographic-Narratives/book-series/WLEN

THERAPY, STAND-UP, AND THE GESTURE OF WRITING
Towards Creative-Relational Inquiry

Jonathan Wyatt

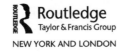

Routledge
Taylor & Francis Group

NEW YORK AND LONDON

First published 2019
by Routledge
52 Vanderbilt Avenue, New York, NY 10017

and by Routledge
2 Park Square, Milton Park, Abingdon, Oxon, OX14 4RN

Routledge is an imprint of the Taylor & Francis Group, an informa business

© 2019 Taylor & Francis

The right of Jonathan Wyatt to be identified as author of this work has been asserted by him in accordance with sections 77 and 78 of the Copyright, Designs and Patents Act 1988.

Library of Congress Cataloging-in-Publication Data
A catalog record for this title has been requested

ISBN: 978-1-138-89762-5 (hbk)
ISBN: 978-1-138-89770-0 (pbk)
ISBN: 978-1-315-17879-0 (ebk)

Typeset in ITC Legacy Serif
by Apex CoVantage, LLC

Printed and bound by CPI Group (UK) Ltd, Croydon, CR0 4YY

To Jamie Brown, 1991–2016

CONTENTS

ACKNOWLEDGEMENTS

This book has been a long-term project (an oh-so-very-long-term project, I hear some murmur) and there are lavish thanks to offer those who have helped it on its way:

It has been invaluable to take chapters in progress to different events over the four years of writing. Knowing each was approaching gave me reason to write. Thank you to Jane Speedy and the Artful Narrative Inquiry Network at Bristol, Ken Gale and the Plymouth Institute of Education, Grace O'Grady and the Department of Education, Maynooth University, the 2017 British Conference of Autoethnography, and the 2017 United Kingdom Council for Psychotherapy Research Conference for invitations to speak; and thank you to all those who attended, asked questions, responded and/or talked with me after. Thanks too to the incomparable Norman Denzin for the continuing wonder that is the annual International Congress of Qualitative Inquiry, where many of these chapters had their first airings.

A number of readers gave me their thoughts and time on parts or all of the manuscript at various points, in particular Tony E. Adams, Dagmar Alexander, Gail Boldt, Liz Bondi, Bronwyn Davies, Ken Gale, Richard Freeman, Hannah Shakespeare and Ron Pelias. Clicking send was always tinged with terror but I knew each would respond with bounty and insight.

Colleagues and students involved in both my academic department (Counselling, Psychotherapy and Applied Social Sciences) and the Centre for Creative-Relational Inquiry at Edinburgh have been an engaged and supportive presence in pushing forward the ideas this book explores. Those conversations on Thursday evenings at Doctors and over coffees at Checkpoint kept lifting me. Thank you.

Liz Bondi, Heather Wilkinson and Alette Willis covered for me as head of department during June and July 2018 as I completed the manuscript. Ah, the space this allowed me. They can only imagine how good that was.

Charlotte Clarke, Head of the School of Health in Social Science: I am full of gratitude for her constant support throughout.

Hannah Shakespeare and Tony E. Adams: publisher and editor extraordinaires, respectively. Thanks to both for their stalwart encouragement and ready advice.

Dave Allison, old friend: for those warm, stimulating, funny discussions over beer and curry when we managed to be in the same city. Like we did at nineteen and will still be doing when we're 80, if we're lucky.

Ken Gale, Bronwyn Davies, Iain MacRury, Ron Pelias, Laurel Richardson, Tami Spry, and Katie Stewart: for reading and responding with endorsements. Such generosity, all. As I write I have no idea what each of them will make of the book or what they will write but, whatever, I owe them coffee/tea/beer/wine, or one of each, at least.

I am indebted to a host of friends, students, colleagues and passing acquaintances for conversations in pubs and cafés, on buses and trains, at comedy shows, conferences, meetings and more, where they pointed me to readings, performers or theory, sent me links, lent me books or were simply interested. Those moments gave me hope. Kat Corbet, Jess Erb, Kate Fox, Jo Hilton, Alecia Jackson, Peter Knox, Lisa Mazzei, Bill McCarty, Alys Mendus, Roberta Mock, Susan Morrison, Robbie Nicol, Seamus Prior, Sophie Tamas, Sarah Truman, Monika Maria Tulismanora—and I know there are others. Thank you, all.

Holly Wyatt and Joe Wyatt, for tolerating being part of this project without complaint. And for being everything they are.

Tess Wyatt: listener, reader, designer. For being here throughout. For making this possible.

Jonathan Wyatt
University of Edinburgh
August 2018

Part 1

Openings[1]

---

1 'Opening' not only as beginning but also as break, as a way to make movement possible, as a signal of the "promise of possibility for difference". Boldt and Leander, "Becoming Through 'the Break'", 2017, 423. Three 'opening' chapters follow.

CHAPTER 1

AN INTRODUCTION

June and July 2018, Edinburgh[2]

THERAPY: KARL

"Time to stop", I say.

"It always comes around so fast, doesn't it?", Karl replies. "No, that's not quite true". He pauses for a moment. "Sometimes it's like we stand still. Like this all stands still".

He begins to rise from his chair, as do I, but, halfway to standing, left hand on the armrest, he freezes, crouched, staring ahead. "Sometimes, here feels like this", he says.

"Thanks for the demo", I laugh.

STAND-UP: SUNDAY 23 OCTOBER 2017,
THE STAND COMEDY CLUB, EDINBURGH

I am standing at the back, a glass of Twister Thistle IPA beside me on the turquoise, distressed shelf, waiting for Fern Brady's show to begin.[3] It is 8.05pm, for an 8.30pm start. The place feels subdued and not yet full. I am on my own in this corner. A man with a beard and jacket has joined me and I appreciate the company, though we haven't spoken. I am not interested in conversation. I have been standing alone here since I arrived. There were seats free but I feel less intrusive being here with my notebook than writing squeezed between others, who would understandably wonder why. It is not an innocent, neutral act to be writing in a comedy club.

WRITING, 20 JUNE 2018, EDINBURGH

Not long now: this book is close to completion, the deadline of 31 July in view. The text has been calling for an introduction and the clarity introductions promise.

The writing-story of this introduction is one characterized by a dynamic of approach and retreat.[4] At times, sentences have formed themselves into definite, purposeful shape, engendering in me a sense of solidity, like pegging the ropes of a tent in a strong wind. In those moments I can stand back and grasp what this book is doing, can see its contours. However, at other times, as with most of my tent-assembling experiences, there have been shaky, fractious moments—maybe it has to be so—and I have had to turn away for a while (to stretch my shoulders and back, to revise a sentence I am not happy with elsewhere, to make coffee) so I can consider how to come back to it differently. You might not hear this movement, this approach and retreat—forth and back, back and forth—in what follows, but it is there, pulsing between the lines.

***

THERAPY, STAND-UP, WRITING

In this book I put therapy and stand-up comedy in circuit with each other, through and with writing, to see what happens. The book, in this sense, is experimental, playful: it is serious play.[5]

The book is not about therapy and stand-up, nor even about writing, for their own sakes, but about what they do together, how they speak to and with each other about, for example, surprise, directness and relationality. The book's heart—heart as rhythm, movement and flux, not heart as static core or centre—is in how, one through and with the other, therapy and stand-up connect with writing as a method of inquiry, engaging and breathing with—and mobilizing—theory throughout.

This theory, these theoretical bodies, these theoretical energies that inform the book, is/are those of Deleuze and Guattari, new materialism (or the new materialisms)[6] and affect theory.[7] Such bodies of theory see affect, for example, not as belonging to one or more individual body but as a "varied, surging capacit[y]" that "catch[es] people up in something that feels like something",[8] a capacity that, in Erin Manning's terms, 'de-phases'[9] in us before moving on elsewhere. Furthermore, from these theoretical perspectives, the 'people', the 'us', are not humanist individual subjects but entities 'intra-acting' with material, human and more-than-human others[10] within a flattened ontology,[11] part of and produced in 'assemblages'[12] of times of day, space, bodies, objects, movement and more.

I say these theoretical bodies and energies 'inform' the book, which suggests passivity on both their part and mine. Instead, I intend 'inform' to work in Erin Manning's active and processual sense of 'in-form' (after Simondon), of being active in, and party to, the book's taking shape.[13] I tussle, I dance, I breathe, with these theories, and they with me; they shape me, they shape this book. As St. Pierre says, theory produces us.[14]

I use 'counselling' and 'therapy' (and counsellor, therapist) interchangeably in the text, with 'therapy' shorthand for 'psychotherapy'. While there are arguments within the field about how counselling and psychotherapy differ, there is much they share.

I began my training as a counsellor in the early 1990s, completing it in 2001 at the Isis Centre, Oxford,[15] my training throughout being *psychodynamic*. Psychodynamic theory and practice are located within the 20th-century psychoanalytic tradition of Freud, Jung, Klein and their successors, and is concerned, for example, with the links between past and present experiences, and with the significance of our unconscious life.

I have long thought of myself as a psychodynamic counsellor, and that continues to be a story I tell, though the label feels slippery and happily complicated. I am influenced by other approaches, like narrative therapy,[16] and over the past ten or more years I have been energized in my life and practice(s), including my therapeutic practice, by the theoretical charge of those I draw from in this book, in particular Deleuze and Guattari. Deleuze and Guattari's work is challenging of psychoanalysis, yet Guattari continued to practise as a psychoanalyst at the innovative La Borde clinic throughout his working life. I embrace Guattari's (and Deleuze and Guattari's) concept of 'the refrain' in relation to therapy in Chapter 5.

I assume throughout the text that counselling is face-to-face, rather than, say, online or by telephone. Similarly, for stand-up, the particular interest of this book is in live performance, where a performer and audience share material(izing) space together, rather than recorded performances I watch or listen to.[17] In both stand-up and therapy, what is crucial for this book's purposes is the immediacy, the here-and-now, flesh-to-flesh presence of bodies in/of rooms; the ebbs and flows of energy, how tension builds and is released: how affect, elusive and mercurial, happens, flows, erupts;[18] how affect—humour, sadness, anger, etc.—arrives in, moves through and changes, becomes, the space. English comedian Ross Noble's comments concerning stand-up's immediacy speak to both stand-up and therapy:

> The joy and the secret of it is in that moment. It is not a passive medium— all the elements must come together, the ideas, the performance and the environment must perfectly align and the comic must merge all of these elements perfectly, controlling and timing everything just right while the audience gets lost in the moment.[19]

Noble does not go far enough here, though. It is not only the audience (and client) but also the performer (and therapist) who needs to allow themselves to become lost.

There are a number of stand-up genres and styles:[20] amongst current, well-known UK-based comics, the likes of Milton Jones work with puns and word-play, others such as Mark Thomas work with big-picture politics and still others, like Michael McIntyre, do 'observational' comedy. The connections I make here are not with these but with the genres of performers such as UK-based North Americans, Reginald D. Hunter and Katherine Ryan, on the one hand, who work with personal and often painful material from their own lives (apparently),[21] and also with the deconstructive, postmodern work of Stewart Lee, whose attention and commentary is as much upon the here-and-now relationship with his audience and his own process as on his show's content.

This is not a pedagogic text about therapy or stand-up. I mostly wear the theoretical and technical complexities of therapeutic practice lightly, aware there is much more to say, understand and explore; nor do I claim expertise as either a comedy connoisseur or performer,[22] knowing many of the form's subtleties and histories pass me by. Nor (my final disclaimer) do I do justice, I know, to the breadth and depth of the scholarly and theoretical literature on each of these sets of practices. Instead, the purpose of this book is to tell their stories, stories of being in the counselling room with clients and of witnessing, and occasionally offering, stand-up performances, seeking for those stories to speak to and with each other, as well as to and with writing and the book's theoretical forces. Writing through such stories enables me to live in and with both therapy and stand-up differently. It is my hope readers also will find this 'diffractive' work—putting one through the other through the other[23]—productive. I hope, too, that my renderings of therapy and stand-up convey the respect and love I have for both the therapeutic and stand-up encounters, and the sense of mystery in what is made possible in both, alongside their inevitable muddle, mess and struggle.

Writing as a Method of Inquiry

Laurel Richardson's proposal in the mid-1990s that writing is a method of inquiry was groundbreaking.[24] Julie White's 2016 volume, *Permission*, explores the influence of Richardson's work over the years since, speaking both from her own experience and through tributes collected from over fifty scholars to how Richardson's writing has inspired and shaped their work.[25] As one such contributor, Larry Russell, writes,

> Many of us write because of [Laurel Richardson]—not writing like her, but writing into the silence at the end of her stories. She invites a level of disclosure found only in old friendships or fine writing. We are drawn into a conversation so faithful to our experience, so intimately radical, that we must carve out new ground to meet her.[26]

The impact of Laurel Richardson's scholarship, and in particular writing-as-inquiry,[27] on qualitative research theorizing and practice has been far-reaching. Radical and provocative, disruptive and generative, writing-as-inquiry continues to open both itself and ourselves as qualitative scholars to new possibilities as we respond to the calls and challenges at the theoretical, methodological, ethical and political edges.

Having made those claims for writing-as-inquiry, and notwithstanding White's book, I would propose there is a 'quietness' to the ways in which Richardson's (and Richardson and St. Pierre's)[28] work on writing-as-inquiry has been taken up. While qualitative research conferences

host special interest groups on other (arguably) closely related methodological approaches like autoethnography and, similarly, journals publish special issues and publishers have book series on such approaches,
only a few of these outlets name writing-as-inquiry as a focus.[29] It is the
collaborative writing initiatives spearheaded by Jane Speedy and the
plentiful collaborative writing assemblages (including mine with Ken
Gale, together and with others) over the years arising out of Speedy's
Narrative Inquiry Centre at Bristol, that I would suggest have taken up
Richardson's proposal that writing is (a method of) inquiry most explicitly and extensively.[30]

I first read and began to write with Laurel Richardson's texts at the
beginning of my doctoral programme at Bristol with Jane Speedy in
February 2004. Ken Gale (who happened to begin the same programme
as well that month) and I began to write together soon after, picking
up on writing-as-inquiry as we brought collaborative writing into conversation with Deleuze and Guattari. Richardson's work has stayed
with us, and with me, since. My contribution to Julie White's *Permission*
reads:

> Laurel Richardson once asked me to read to her. Discovering writing
> changed my life (not always for the better). It wasn't just Laurel. There were
> other factors (where I was in my life, the loss of my father, a supportive
> workplace) and other people (some who knew it, some who didn't—I'm
> not sure which category applies to Laurel). Circumstances, people, places,
> time, even the stars perhaps, all aligned and I discovered writing. Nor was
> it about before or after, a turning point, a Damascene moment. That's not
> how it was, nor how Laurel would want it. But there was this one moment
> in May 2007, one I remember, whatever claim I might not make for it. There
> had been other encounters with Laurel, significant in their way, like read-
> ing *Fields of Play*,[31] where she took me (and countless others) on her aca-
> demic voyage; and, meanwhile, showed me how and what it was possible to
> write. There was "Writing as Method of Inquiry" in the 1994 and 2005 Sage
> Handbooks, and 'Evaluating Ethnography' in a 2000 [important][32] special
> issue of *Qualitative Inquiry*. I had already found her, drawn from her, talked
> with her (not that she had been aware), talked about her (ditto). Yes, she
> was already there; here. But this moment, this series of moments, is what
> I remember most. It was nothing grand. It was a gesture of interest and
> generosity on her part, an unnecessary gift: She asked me to read to her a

story I'd written. We were at a conference. Earlier, I had been in a workshop
with Laurel. Others had read their work and I chose not to. That evening—
no, it must have been the next day, or the day after that; some years on, I've
lost the sequence. One evening, let's say, at the conference cookout, I was
standing with friends at a table. Laurel Richardson approached, joined our
conversation, and later asked me to read to her the writing I hadn't shared
at the workshop. I did and she listened, as did the others (what choice did
they have?); and the conversations continued. That was it, in a way. No eval-
uative discussion, no praise, no critique, just listening; but the story found
a life in a collaborative writing project with others, two of whom were at our
table that evening. And I found a life in this story: Laurel listening to my
writing. It was nothing much, and it was everything.[33]

That text from *Permission* described my encounter with Laurel Richardson and her work. In what follows in this book I carry with me others'
scholarship on writing and/as inquiry. I carry with me Ron Pelias' (and
others') *performative writing*, writing that "aims to keep the complexities
of human experience intact, to place the ache back in scholars' abstrac-
tions";[34] a writing that does;[35] a writing that aspires to intervene in the
everyday of the personal/social/political; a writing that, as Della Pollock
would put it, is *nervous*: "unable to settle into a clear, linear, course, neither willing nor able to stop moving, restless, transient and transitive,
traversing spatial and temporal borders".[36] I carry Deleuze—"to write is
to trace lines of flight"[37]—and I carry Hélène Cixous, whose writing as
'gesture', is conveyed in this book's title.[38]

My intention in this sole-authored book (sole-authored, yet always
collaboratively written, as Speedy would argue[39]) is to engage, engage
with, and put to work, the claims Richardson, Pelias, Pollock, Deleuze,
Cixous and others make for writing, as I move between therapy and
stand-up and as I activate the concept of *creative-relational inquiry*.

CREATIVE-RELATIONAL INQUIRY

In late afternoon on Thursday 12 October 2017, we launched the *Centre
for Creative-Relational Inquiry* (CCRI, or Sea Cry) in Edinburgh.[40] The rain
fell, but from the top floor of the Edinburgh College of Art you could
still make out Edinburgh castle to the north on its volcanic perch, its
dim lights glistening. About thirty people attended the launch event,

both from within and beyond the university: researchers, performers, artists, writers, therapists, policy makers; some local, some from further afield (one from Toronto, via Manchester).

Like the rounded shape of a shell you happen upon as your bare foot presses the damp sand, the notion of *creative-relational inquiry* emerged while walking on a beach in Cornwall in summer, 2016. It was Saturday 25 June. I remember: it was two days after the UK had voted to leave the European Union and we were mourning. The beach was the three-mile sweep of Whitsand Bay on Cornwall's southern coast. We were staying with Ken Gale, who lives nearby.

For months I had been writing, dreaming and talking with friends and colleagues, about the new research centre; about why it was needed and what it could do. I had played around with names. In early drafts I had called the centre, the *Centre for Transformative Inquiry* (too clichéd), the *Centre for Qualitative Inquiry* (too broad), and the *Centre for Transformative Qualitative Inquiry* (too both). The notion of 'centre' was and remains problematic, in its implications of stasis and hierarchy (as if it were something like a seat of government), but there did not seem an alternative, not least because of the designation of 'centres' within my university.

"Walking, dancing, pleasure: these accompany the poetic act", writes Hélène Cixous.[41] It is not only about being at your desk in the back room typing, or sitting in the nook of your favourite café with your notebook open, pen poised. Sometimes you need to move, or move differently. "Walking-writing is a thinking-in-movement", write Springgay and Truman. I walked, barefoot on the summer sand, most likely not aware I was 'thinking' about this imagined centre but, for sure, aware of my sadness for my country, and there was *creative-relational inquiry*.

The name survived further drafts and comments from colleagues. I found the Brian Massumi chapter where he uses the term 'creative-relational',[42] and, finalizing the title for this book around that time in 2016, took the risk of using creative-relational inquiry as its framing concept. I wanted to use this book to explore the proposition of 'creative-relational inquiry', seeking to open up its possibilities through therapy, stand-up and writing-as-inquiry; to put this new and raw concept to work and see where it might take us.[43] The series of 'Intervals' in the book, in particular, pushes at these possibilities.

AN OVERVIEW OF *THERAPY*, *STAND-UP*,
AND THE *GESTURE* OF *WRITING*

For four years I have been carrying versions of chapters of *Therapy, Stand-Up, and the Gesture of Writing* to various events, bringing the text to some sort of life in seminar rooms and conference spaces. When I now bring this book's imagined reader to life at their desks or in their living rooms, in airport lounges, in libraries, or wherever, it is similar audiences I sense I am writing/reading to: researcher-writer-scholars who share an interest in storied, performative and embodied scholarship;[44] those seeking ways in which they might bring current—and complex— theories to bear upon their research practices; and counselling and psychotherapy practitioner-researchers, and those in related fields (e.g. social workers, educators), who are looking for fresh ways to undertake and theorize their inquiries. My hope is there will be something here for each of these.

What follows works with and at the connections between therapy, stand-up and writing. I use the one to riff off the other, the one to provide insight into the other, the one to diffract through the other. At times, how they meet, how they encounter each other, is explicit, at others implicit. I tell stories and vignettes of and from the live work of a few well-known comics (well-known in the UK, at least) but more from the immediacy of routine nightly shows and the witnessing of often local, unknown performers at Edinburgh's comedy clubs and other venues. I bring into play my own ventures into stand-up performance.

Alongside—imbricated with—such tales, the book draws from my work as a therapist. The stories and vignettes of my work with one particular client, Karl, as we talk together in room 4 on Tuesday evenings at the counselling agency where I practise, run throughout the book.[45] I also feature work with occasional other clients.

I offer these stories of stand-up and therapy alongside those stories and poems of the everyday profound of writing-as-inquiry—including working, travelling, visiting my mother, mourning my late father and more—suggesting how each (therapy, stand-up and writing) has echoes of the other. And through bringing these into conversation with each other I inquire into how this diffractive process does productive theoretical work with Deleuze and Guattari, new materialism and affect theory as the text pushes and pulls at a conceptualizing and embodying of *creative-relational inquiry*.

***

THERAPY: KARL

"Thanks for the demo", I laugh.

"Not at all". Karl picks up his coat and bag.

I open the door for us to leave, but he hesitates on his way out: "Thinking about it, this"—gesturing back towards the room—"never feels frozen. 'Standing still', I said, but what I did was to freeze. Being still isn't the same as being frozen. Something happens in stillness".

"Yes, sure".

STAND-UP: SUNDAY 23 OCTOBER 2017, THE STAND COMEDY CLUB, EDINBURGH

I notice the mural behind the stage. It is an image of a boy, perhaps eight or nine years old. He is dressed as a cowboy, with a pale cowboy hat, brown neckerchief, blue and grey check shirt and yellow waistcoat. In his left hand he holds a toy pistol to his temple. He smiles: a thin, resigned, fuck-it smile. He in turn is, it seems, on stage, the shadow of arm and pistol on the dark wall behind him.

We are playing, the image seems to suggest through the picture of the child in fancy-dress. This is an act, and we are all playing, having fun, but the shadow suggests something more serious. We are playing with life and death.

The mural seems to be asking, what is really at stake?

WRITING, 28 JUNE 2018

It is all but done, this introduction, this one way into the book. Not the only way to begin, but it has been a way for me as writer to loop back into what follows. Meanwhile, I have been writing into other sections of the book, re-ordering, cutting, re-phrasing, and now, this Thursday morning—a high summer's day that is calling for sun screen and ice cream—I have returned here. I will return again to re-read and to adjust but I sense it is all but there, ropes pegged and taut.

NOTES

2 Chapters, and some sections within chapters, indicate dates and places of the writing, suggesting the writing is situated, that it is a view from somewhere. Yet this is complicated by my having begun writing a chapter at one time and place, including drawing from earlier writing (as in the first stand-up entry on this page, which is from notes made at an event in 2017), and then often revising a chapter on a number of occasions, with those returns mostly remaining implicit. The book does not follow through chronologically but moves between times, working less with what Deleuze would call *chronos*—linear, sequential time—and more with *aiôn*, "time as potentiality, the sense in which time cannot be grasped because it is always simultaneously moving into the past and the future". Boldt and Leander, "Becoming Through 'the Break' ", 2017, 418. See Deleuze, *Logic of Sense*, 1990.

3 *Male Comedienne.*

4 Richardson, *Fields of Play*, 1997. Laurel Richardson's book contains papers and essays, written over a ten-year period, alongside stories about how they came to be written, their 'writing-stories'. Writing-stories do political work in how they situate and position the writer: "Writing is demystified, writing strategies are shared, and the field is unbounded", 3.

5 I am drawing upon Jasmine Ulmer here: "I find that playful writing can be helpful when it provides the time and space to distil what is important and is at stake. Play can be serious". Ulmer, "Composing Techniques", 2017, 7.

6 Coole and Frost, *New Materialisms*, 2010; St. Pierre, Jackson and Mazzei, "New Empiricisms and New Materialisms", 2016. Coole and Frost pluralize 'new materialisms' in order to acknowledge the field's various and varying initiatives.

7 e.g. Gregg and Seigworth, *The Affect Theory Reader*, 2010. However, affect *theory*, as a term, is problematic. It is not a term Deleuze and Guattari use, for example. They talk of *affect*. Affect *theory* is perhaps suggestive of abstraction.

8 Stewart, *Ordinary Affects*, 2007, 1.

9 Manning, *Always More Than One*, 2013.

10 Barad, *Meeting the Universe Halfway*, 2007.

11 'Flattened ontology': in other words, there is no hierarchy of being, no one element (in that word's colloquial, not scientific, sense) of life (the universe and everything) that has precedence over another or is ever able to stand outside, or above, another. Everything is in it together: "[T]hings and people, social and natural entities, institutions and microbes are treated as analytically symmetrical". Jenson, "A Nonhumanist Disposition", 2004, 256.

12 Deleuze and Guattari, *A Thousand Plateaus*, 2004.

13 Manning, *Always More Than One*, 2013.

14 St. Pierre, "The Posts Continue", 2013

15 The wonderful Isis Centre was the first 'walk-in' NHS counselling service in

the UK, established in large part through the vision and energy of Dr Peter Agulnik, whom I was lucky to have as my clinical supervisor for two years.

16 e.g. White, *Reflections on Narrative Practice*, 2000.

17 There is one exception to this. I refer to listening to Reginald D. Hunter's audio recording of a Reginald D. Hunter performance in Chapter 3.

18 Stewart, *Ordinary Affects*, 2007.

19 Double, *Getting the Joke*, 2013, x.

20 Double.

21 Less the case with Ryan's more recent work. It is her performances of around 2014 that I am thinking of here. See Chapter 3.

22 Chapter 12 will testify to the latter.

23 I am drawing upon Karen Barad (and Donna Haraway) in working with the concept of 'diffraction': "A diffractive methodology seeks to work constructively and deconstructively (not destructively) in making new patterns of understanding-becoming". Barad, "Diffracting Diffraction", 2014, 187n. See also Chapter 11.

24 Richardson, "Writing: A Method of Inquiry", 1994 and 2000. Richardson notes, however, that writers have long known of writing's heuristic power. It was in the academy, or the social sciences at least, that writing had become reduced to the instrumental function of 'writing up'.

25 White, *Permission*, 2016.

26 White, 15.

27 I use this term because it is snappier than 'writing as a method of inquiry', and to challenge the implicit reductiveness of writing as (only) 'method'. See Interval: Towards Creative-Relational Inquiry (1).

28 Richardson and St. Pierre, "Writing: A Method of Inquiry", 2005, 2017.

29 See the programmes, for example, for recent iterations of the International and European Congresses of Qualitative Inquiry.

30 Such collaborative writing assemblages include Speedy *et al.*, "Encountering Gerald", 2010; Gale *et al.*, "Collaborative Writing in Real Time", 2012; etc. The Narrative Inquiry Centre is now the Arts-informed Narrative Inquiry Network (ANINET), University of Bristol. (The web link is too long to include here but is easily searchable.)

31 Richardson, *Fields of Play*, 1997.

32 I used the gendered, sexist term, 'seminal', in the original so have replaced it here.

33 White, *Permission*, 2016, 82–3.

34 Pelias, "Performative Writing as Scholarship", 2005.

35 Gale, *Madness as Methodology*, 2018.

36 Pollock, "Performing Writing", 1998.

37 Deleuze and Parnet, *Dialogues II*, 2002, 32.

38 See Chapter 2.

39 "[A]ll writing is collaborative, insofar as all writing is an *embodied and imagined* accumulation of *selves and stories*", Speedy, "Collaborative Writing and Ethical Know-how", 2012, 355. Emphasis in the original.

40 https://www.ed.ac.uk/health/research/ccri

41 Cixous, 1994, p. 202.

42 See Chapter Interval: Towards Creative-Relational Inquiry (1): Take It to Heart.

43 I use 'proposition' in Manning and Massumi's sense: "Propositions are not intended as a set of directions or rules that contain and control movement, but as prompts for further experimentation and thought". Springgay and Truman, *Walking Methodologies*, 2018, 14. See Manning and Massumi, *Thought in the Act*, 2014.

44 See note 34 of Interval: Towards Creative-Relational Inquiry (2): The Problem and Promise of the Personal.

45 The counselling agency is *The PF Counselling Service*, a well-established and respected counselling service in south Edinburgh. www.pfcounselling.org.uk/ I am grateful to Alison Hampton, The PF's manager, for her support for this project. My work with Karl is offered not as a 'clinical case study', with the implication that it is illustrative of an aspect of therapeutic theory or practice. Instead, Karl is an encounter: "something that happens in between and takes on its own direction", Jackson, "Thinking Without Method", 2017, 670.

CHAPTER 2

SOMETHING MIGHT HAPPEN

July 2014, Montjaux

This chapter was written at the beginning of the process of writing this book in 2014. I have returned to it, as I have read and written further, but much of it is as it was handwritten in my journal at the time. It is, in a sense, another introduction to the book, a writing-story about the beginning of writing.

MONDAY 21 JULY 2014

Step inside the white chalk circle: everything is possible.

That first sentence matters. *Step inside the white chalk circle: everything is possible.* First impressions. How the sentence feels on the flesh: whether it caresses or strikes, or both; whether it feels cool to the touch or warming, or both: a paradox, an oxymoron. What its textures do, the colours it evokes, the sounds it makes. The hollows it forms in the skin. Where it leaves the reader. First impressions.

That first sentence matters, but I know it can't ever be right. It can't ever do all I want it to. It's asking too much, though first sentences can do great work. Think of first lines: Austen, Tolstoy, Orwell. This one, a favourite, from Iain Banks: "It was the day my grandmother exploded".[46] There's the reader's surprise and laughter, and our sense of horror; and we infer love, perhaps (though not all grandmothers are loved); loss too, we assume, though we don't know and don't feel that yet, not in those first moments, not when we're laughing.

Step inside the white chalk circle: everything is possible.

The first sentence matters, but maybe it matters only as much as any other. One will follow another, then another. I say, 'sentence', but that's too neutral. "Step inside". It's a command. Or you could read it as an invitation, an enticement. A promise follows. "Everything is possible". A promise you may or may not trust, or want; a promise I can never keep. A promise we can never realize, never see, never know; a promise that could send us over, send us mad. Send us to despair: at what we can't see, can't find, what isn't there; at what we can never reach.

But perhaps stepping inside is still worth the risk.

Step inside the white chalk circle. Something might happen. Something might be possible.

Yes, let's live with that, for now. Step inside the white chalk circle. Something might happen. Something might be possible.

***

I have begun writing on a narrow first floor blue metal balcony in Montjaux, in the Aveyron region of southern France, one early evening in July. I can hear a fly as it darts above me, near the gutter, and in the distance the sound of a tractor. I look up and I can see the tractor skirting a strip of ploughed field on the side of the steep hill to my left in the middle distance.

We are here earlier in the summer than usual and there is an unfamiliar luxuriance in everything, the life not yet burnt from a lush land. By the roadside below, a cluster of fuchsia hollyhocks stand six feet tall, a friendly greeting as cars approach the village.

I am face on to a strong breeze from the southwest; clumps of cloud approach underneath an apparently static, uniform, grey sky.

Beginning this book in this place feels right. It's where we come each summer to replenish spent reserves. It's the distance we travel to stop and think. It's where I come to read, or read differently; and to write— notes and fragments, and handwritten drafts in a notebook. I always imagine I will read more and write more than I ever do, but still, something different happens, something gets done. Here is where my contributions to various, mostly collaborative, texts have taken shape over the years. It is where I have felt my writing companions most present, as if, with the clutter of everyday life removed, or with a different clutter, there is space for others. I have been able to pen for co-authors apparently inconsequential stories about sheep and the sounds of French being spoken near me in cafés.[47] I have been able to tell stories of this place and our days here and find my 'writing others' close by. So here, now, I am using this balcony, this wind, these pale, rough stone walls beside me, to find a way to begin to write again, to search again. Beyond this, me, here, now, to someone(s), something(s), somewhere else.

***

On the balcony[48]

sun-skin-hot on iron-cast balcony-blue
butterflies swirldancing, gathering-scattering
cicadas calling, birds sing-beckoning
trees swaying—gentle, gentle—
forth back back-forth trees-swaying

fly-restless-hand-sweep, from balcony-blue
the rolling world is far-as-scanning-eye greening, greening
yellow-punctuated lavender-rupted
greening, greening—ah, but there—
one browning, folding field-earth

on iron-cast balcony-blue, breathing-body
soar-surfing the breezing air
keening-sinew-bones-blood
melting into the—taken by the—
falling-rising rise-fall of the not-yet might-be

***

This afternoon I had the river to myself. We drove from the village in sunlight down the hill and into a gathering darkness. Drops began to fall on the windscreen five minutes from the riverside and by the time we parked under the trees the intense burst of rain was at its peak. Tess had her book and I sat watching the assault on the cloudy emerald surface of the slow-moving water.

The storm passed. This was to be my first swim of the summer and I was not feeling bold, so I waited in the car. When I glimpsed blue sky above the ridge it was time to move. I got out, ran down the grass slope to the river edge, trod warily onto the rocks, and eased in, kicking to the centre of the broad, sluggish river, but no further. Being alone I felt cautious and vulnerable. I front-crawled upstream, attempting to get my breathing regular and sustainable, but couldn't. So I floated back downstream, and paused, treading water.

Treading water; treading words; words at feet and fingers, pawing just to stay still; words on the surface passing as I watched; a dream. Last night's dreams. I had begun writing before I went to bed, just a paragraph. In between my many wakeful moments in the night this book seemed to take shape. In my dreaming, chapters were written and sequenced, the writing endeavour purposeful and gathering momentum, but then I would wake and know nothing was yet done. The satisfaction of having started, however, remained in those dark hours as another thunderstorm passed. A book, any book, has to be started.

The sun has left the hills to the east. I have a beer in my hand. This is where I'm beginning, in this quiet, distant world, on this few square feet of balcony. I have left in Edinburgh a pile of tasks and concerns that need attending to (I am head of my university department: who is going to teach that course? What rooms will we be allocated? When will we know? And so on); and there are complex decisions to be made with my family in Godalming, south-east England, concerning my mother's care. How is it that only a matter of months ago she was in her own home making major financial and life decisions with authority and now she is uncertain and dependent? How has that happened so fast? Where has she gone?

And beyond—beyond Edinburgh, beyond Godalming, beyond Montjaux—the world is in turmoil, Flight M17 shot from the sky on Thursday and Gaza ablaze.

What kind of an act, then, is writing? (I leave that question mark on the page, hesitate and begin the opening bracket, shaping its arc on the third line of my notebook.) It has to be something. It is a "gesture of love", says Hélène Cixous.[49] "*The gesture*", she adds, the italics—the emphasis—her own, asserting that "this is the one and only gesture, readers". Writing is fragile but not futile; gesture does not carry the meaning of tokenism here. Writing is the movement we make towards the other and towards the world. No, no, that—'towards'—is not right, will not do, because the separation it implies—between me, you, other, world—does not hold.[50]

19

Writing is the movement, the gesture, *of* the world, *of* the other (my emphasis this time), in its "in/determinacy" and its "always already opening up-to-come".[51] Writing is an act of resistance to the pressure to stay silent, to do nothing. A small act of activism.[52]

This is a claim of and for this book, that writing matters, can make a difference; and that writing, in particular about therapy and stand-up, speaks to and of a world beyond itself; it connects. Connects theory and therapy, loving and losing, laughing and crying. A claim that if we step inside the white chalk circle, if we take the risk, if we write, work, live, in the white chalk circle, then *something might happen*.

The white chalk circle: British stand-up performer, Stewart Lee, tells the story of how, one summer in rural France in an ancient village—much like Montjaux, I imagine, though he does not specify where it is—he followed a troupe of drama student performers staging a performance of a mediaeval practice whereby those who at the time would have been the outcasts of mediaeval French society, the *bouffons* (the 'mad', the 'fools', those who might now be ascribed the label 'mentally ill'), were, for a day, given the freedom of the village. He was witnessing this annual event, the students moving apparently at random from place to place within the village, to mark this one day in the year when the village *bouffons*, rather than being kept out of sight and sound, which was the case the rest of the year, were given licence to roam at will within the village, saying and doing whatever they wished.

Lee writes how, when the performers reached the village church (Roman Catholic, of course), they drew a rough circle in chalk on the paving stones of the square outside. When, and only when, they entered the circle, the *bouffons* could say whatever they wished, even (especially) about the Church, about God, about the Virgin Mary. Whatever was taboo to say against religion was permissible within the ragged white chalk circle.

Lee was astonished. He writes:

> I was thrilled, not in some adolescent way, about to enjoy a gratuitous mockery of religion, but because something essential about what stand-up was had suddenly, by association, become clear. The bouffons were in a charmed circle, perhaps under the protection of serpents, in a sacred and clearly delineated space where they were free to work their magic without interference. The director of *The Aristocrats*, Paul Provenza, once told me he saw the stage of a stand-up club as a giant pair of inverted commas, framing

the performer, saying "what is being said here is only being said, not actually done, so judge it accordingly". Could there be any clearer image for the special privileges of the comedian than this moment, where the clowns marked out their own unassailable territory in the very shadow of the church, the great forbidder that binds with briars our joys and desires?[53]

Step inside the white chalk circle. Something might happen. Something might be possible.

On his return to his own performances, Lee subsequently began his sets by coming on stage and, without explanation to puzzled audiences, drawing a circle in white chalk around him.

When I consider these practices—the *bouffons* and Stewart Lee creating their space to give voice to what is impermissible—I hear them speak on behalf of us all and our yearning for what we all would like to say if only we could allow ourselves to. Our desire to find the "language of the unsayable".[54]

Step inside the white chalk circle. Something might happen. Something might be possible.

Something—or anything—might be possible on the stand-up stage; and something—anything—might be possible on the therapeutic 'stage'. I collect my client from a waiting room on a Tuesday evening at the voluntary agency where I practise. We walk along a pale blue-carpeted corridor, which turns ninety degrees left towards the room I use, room 4, the final room on the right. I lead, my client follows. During the walk my client and I tend not to speak. I prefer it that way. The corridor is an informal space, somewhere only small talk or conversations about the weather are possible, and I don't want that. I don't want to 'chat'. I enter the room first, hold open the door, say my first word, 'Welcome', and we sit in chairs facing each other. There's a side-table between us to one side, on which rests a lamp, tissues, a small rectangular vase of artificial purple and yellow flowers, and a clock. I have my back to the door. There's a window to my left, which I open when clients go and close when the next one arrives. The room always seems too full when we finish.

Coats off, bags on the floor, seated, we begin. Somewhere. Sometimes there's silence; sometimes Karl knows where he wants to start. He has thought on the way here and decided. At others, he opens with "I don't know what I want to talk about today", and we go from there. Either way, we don't know what will take place, where the fifty minutes will go. Something might happen. It is not inevitable, and often apparently nothing happens. This may be the case if I am pre-occupied, perhaps, with the day's events at the university, or worried about my mother, or hungry; or if he is needing to retreat or is distracted or himself pre-occupied; or, to be more precise, if there is some dynamic, some quality of the *haecceity*,[55] the 'this-ness', of the room, the dynamic within and between us and within and between us and the room, the weather, the time of day, and more. But sometimes we stay open. We stay open to what might happen, though the something that might happen might be nothing, a nothing that's needed in that moment. It might be something of nothing. The giant inverted commas bracket us, caress us, and what gets said and done—or just sensed, or held—may not have been ever said and done before, or not said and done in this particular way, and here, in this non-descript room on a Tuesday evening, something becomes possible that would not have been possible anywhere, or anytime, else. Something (or/of nothing) happens.

It is not as Paul Provenza would have it when he claims to Stewart Lee, that "what is being said here is only being said, not actually done, so judge it accordingly",[56] because there is action in the speaking. Speech *acts*, as Austin might put it.[57] Something does happen. In fact, surely Provenza is mistaken in the case of stand-up too. Something is happening there too. It's not just 'joking', it's not just 'pretend'. Something happens.

As Lee watched the *bouffons'* show, it was not only the chalk circle as metaphor that appealed to him but its physical, spatial and material implications:

> [A]s well as the supposed intellectual theory behind the bouffons' show, the spatial relations of the performance also excited me. Like the Native American Pueblo clowns of the Hopi, the Zuni and the Tewa, of whom I had read much but never been fortunate enough to see, even these drama-student bouffons broke through the safety barriers between audience and performer, using the whole village as their stage. You never knew where they were coming from next. Because they were actors, not the anointed clown mystics of the Hopi or the genuine outcasts the medieval French bouffons would have been, it never felt truly dangerous, but the performance did have a relationship, I realised, with moments when I'd seen performers closer to home blur the edge of the space.[58]

In my counselling room, the protagonists are not 'actors' as Lee defines the performers he witnessed. They are 'themselves': their own lives are at stake or, at least, their own *living* is at stake, and in that sense the work is dangerous. It matters. However, as Lee says, there remains an edge to stand-up performance too: there is something at stake there, whatever the 'pretence'. When Lee leaves the stage during the heart of his 2010 show, *If you want a milder comedian please ask for one*, he keeps talking to the audience, apparently angry and disappointed with and cheated by life (this being the theme of this part of the show), berating the intellectual theft by a cider company of a long-established stock phrase within his family of origin (trust me, it made sense at the time). Lee runs along the corridors at the back of the stage, out and up the stairs before re-appearing amongst the audience in the lower circle, still talking, still angry, still ranting, still in despair. Something *is* at stake. Anxiety courses through the theatre. Lee is breaking rules. The anxiety is accompanied by excitement and laughter, but there is risk. What will he do next? Is he ok? As he himself acknowledges in the here and now, the audience is wondering: "Is he. . .? Has he. . .? No, we know what this is. . . . Don't we? But . . . is this some kind of breakdown?" Even as we know he is fine, that this is part of the act, the point is that his performance *affects* the audience in multiple, complex ways. There is jeopardy; something happens.

TUESDAY 22 JULY 2014

I meet writing at the appointed time. My appointed time here today is in the late afternoon on the navy blue wrought-iron balcony, now in shadow.

The far side of the valley is sunlit, its ridge appearing level with me as I sit in the creaking faded canvas chair. Above the ridge in the far distance the seven masts of the magnificent *Viaduc de Millau* appear, like slim rockets ready to launch. I can only see the tips of most of the masts, but the ridge of hills falls to reveal the bodies in full of the two to the far right and the road deck between them, as if those two alone carry its weight.

It is warm enough to sit outside but only just. This morning we sat in the warmth of a summer's day; this evening we are back to late Spring. I am wrapped up. A small child and her mother walk along the narrow road that runs below. They are talking; the child carries a bucket of stones. The mother and child don't look up as they pass underneath and I do not greet them. A fly—a different one, I presume—walks on my page and along my right index finger before leaving, only to return a moment later, higher up my arm. There are more flies than usual this year.

Cixous would be with me in seeing writing itself as a charmed circle. She would see writing this book, this inquiry into how therapy and stand-up meet, as being an adventure. "Writing: touching the mystery", she says, "delicately, with the tips of the words, trying not to crush it, in order to un-lie".[59] Again, as with stand-up and therapy, this is not inevitable, but writing-as-inquiry can touch the mystery.

Cixous would say to Lee as he draws the chalk on the stage flooring, and to the therapist and his client as he holds open the door to room 4 after the corridor walk, and to the writer on this blue balcony: yes, there is the potential for mystery. Take the risk. Make the gesture. Something might happen.

THURSDAY 24 JULY 2014

After yesterday's gleaming day, this morning is overcast and grey. We heard thunder earlier, while our day was still dry, but now that the rain has begun there is only the persistent drip onto the balcony and the pattering on the roof. I'm in shorts and T-shirt, as if willing the sun to return. I may have to give in and find warmer clothes but for now I feel stubborn and sit indoors with the windows onto the balcony open. It *will* be summer. It *will* be July. It *will* be my summer holiday.

My father never knew this place. Tess and I came here with the kids while he was still alive but it would never have suited him, with the steep stairs in the house and the hills all around (he had one leg affected by polio at 19, and Parkinson's Disease from his late fifties), and the long drive would have been too much. When he was younger, he might have managed and enjoyed it all, especially the solitude.

He is with me through these troubled weeks as we seek to work out how best to support Mum and her move into residential care. There is tension between the three of us, the siblings, and we sometimes each invoke our father—"It (*whatever 'it' may be*) is (*or is not*) what Dad would have wanted"—and position him on our respective side of the argument. The cracks between us open as the issue of what she can afford dominates our conversations, and our father's name is reached for in an attempt to draw us together. He would be sad, I imagine. There I go again.

He was where this all began, ten years ago. He was who I wrote for, who I wrote about. His stories drew me to writing, helped me to begin to think of myself as a writer. His loss prompted me to think with him as I wrote about my therapeutic practice.[60] "There is a time in life when you expect the world to be always full of new things", writes Helen MacDonald,

> [a]nd then comes a day when you realise that is not how it will be at all. You see that life will become a thing made of holes. Absences. Losses. Things that were there and are no longer. And you realise, too, that you have to grow around and between the gaps, though you can put your hand out to where things were and feel that tense, shining dullness of the space where the memories are.[61]

Writing is finding a way around and between the gaps, a gesture towards where things were, into the dullness of absence. He, his absence, is why I am here and why this book is happening. He finds his way into therapy, into stand-up and into writing, and the spaces between them all.

SUNDAY 27 JULY 2014

This morning's swim was special. The cool of the water held me close and I paused to hear the wind and take in the verdant green of the surrounding hills. Dad—and I feel confident of this claim—would have enjoyed the swimming here in the early mornings, with the empty river-bank and no one to stare at his leg as he eased himself in, but he always preferred the sea, the way the waves lifted him and created lightness in his body.

I feel sadness. The conflicts within my family kept me awake for over three hours last night. I read a detective novel set in Edinburgh and both missed the place that is now home and felt nostalgic for Abingdon, where, until a year ago, we had lived for twenty-five years.[62] I drafted an email to my siblings, in despair and anger, and sent it to myself. Eased by the writing, I was able to sleep, though not fully. Not well. So today I have been sluggish and bad company and out of touch with this writing until now, when, drying in the late afternoon sun and the cicadas lively to my left, I am here again keeping my appointment with this book, trying to work my way further into its beginning, as the breeze touches my skin and I notice I am alive.

Tuesday 29 July 2014

We leave for home tomorrow. Today has been cold and intermittently damp. I have worn two layers and have only been outside to venture for a slow and tentative run down to the next village, Marzials, looping past the 15th-century church and back up the steep hill the other side, before traversing the side of the mountain back to the house. I paused often on the climb. I am not as fit as I'd hoped.

As she prepares for her move my mother is spending her final weeks at home sifting and sorting her possessions. Over the phone this morning she told me she was looking at the various books and journal issues I've given her to read over the years. "I'll give you them back", she declared. "I don't understand them so there's no point keeping them. But", she hesitated, "there's one I might keep". She didn't tell me which.

I open the low, narrow doors onto the balcony, and step out into the gloom. I can see across the roof of the cloud nestling in the valley just the tips of all seven viaduct masts, their lights blinking red as the day darkens. I stand and listen. I can hear, but not see, the sheep in the steepling field to my left, by the bell that one of them carries. There are no cicadas.

In the morning we will finish cleaning the house, pack up the hire car, and drive the ninety minutes to the airport. By tomorrow evening we will be home, all being well. I will be back at the university on Thursday and will resume seeing counselling clients next week. I will go to stand-up gigs. I will keep writing; I will keep making the gesture, keep working away at where this might lead.

Step with me into the white chalk circle. Something might happen.

Notes

46 Banks, *The Crow Road*, 1992, 3.

47 Wyatt *et al.*, *Deleuze and Collaborative Writing*, 2011.

48 I use poetic writing on occasions in this book with the intention of making language work harder, or work differently at least; and, at times, like here, as an attempt to convey the vibrancy of matter, as Jane Bennett would put it. Bennett talks about the poetry of Walt Whitman, which she is drawn to for its capacity to

express materialism. It "pushes [her] to turn to the bodies that are words". Watson, "Eco-Sensibilities", 2013, 158. See Bennett, *Vibrant Matter*, 2010.

49 Cixous, *Coming to Writing*, 1991, 42.

50 See Barad, *Meeting the Universe Halfway*, 2007; Barad, "Diffracting Diffraction", 2014.

51 Barad, "Diffracting Diffraction", 2014, 178.

52 Madison, *Acts of Activisim*, 2010.

53 Lee, *How I Escaped My Certain Fate*, 2010, 150. There is link here also to Huizinga's proposal that all play takes place within a 'magic circle', a "temporary [world] within the ordinary world, dedicated to the performance of an act apart". Huizinga, *Homo Ludens*, 2002, 10.

54 Rogers *et al.*, "An Interpretive Poetics of Languages of the Unsayable", 1999.

55 Deleuze and Guattari, *A Thousand Plateaus*, 2004.

56 Lee, *How I Escaped My Certain Fate*, 2010, 150.

57 Austin, *How To Do Things With Words*, 1962.

58 Lee, *How I Escaped My Certain Fate*, 2010, 151.

59 Cixous, *Coming to Writing*, 1991, 134.

60 Wyatt, "A Gentle Going", 2005; "No Longer Loss", 2008; etc.

61 MacDonald, *H is for Hawk*, 2014, 171.

62 See Wyatt and Wyatt, "(Be)Coming Home", 2015.

CHAPTER 3

ALWAYS MORE

Autumn 2014, Edinburgh

I began this chapter soon after the Edinburgh Fringe festival in August 2014, having been swept away at stand-up events that month: it was how performers covered their personal-political ground; it was the echoes of therapeutic encounters in the stories they told, and the sleek crafting of their visceral writing. In this chapter I bring the reader further into the book, developing its premise and inquiring into how stories of therapy, stand-up, and writing—and everyday living—are interwoven. I write of and between Karl (my client), my mother and three stand-up performances I witnessed that August (plus a fourth I listened to).

WRITING

I sit alone at a café on George Street, outside, which would be surprising enough in Scotland in July let alone October. The nearby statue of George IV stands aloof amongst the passing shopping hordes.

I'm working my way into the connections and slippages between therapy, stand-up comedy and writing-as-inquiry: how some stand-up, like writing-as-inquiry, works between the personal, the cultural and the political;[63] how stand-up offers embodied texts that take us through and into and back from performers' worlds and leave us affected and changed;[64] and how stand-up, like writing-as-inquiry, sometimes works through and with material that is also the 'stuff' of therapy.[65] My desire is to enquire into how therapy, stand-up, and writing concern the playful, the watchful, and the poignant, in circuit with each other, fluid and dynamic between therapist and client, performer and audience, writer and the page and the reader, enmeshed within spaces and places, and times of day; how all three attend to the intimate in this material, affective world.

A hen party lurches by. The 'hen' approaches with a bucket, calling,

"A pound for a kiss?" and stands waiting. It's more a demand than a request. Her chicks raise a cheer.

"I don't have a pound", I lie. She tilts her head to one side, places a hand on her hip and intones "Well, how much have you got?" to a chorus of "Oooooo!" from her chicks. So, I find a coin, a pound, drop it in the bucket and we exchange a peck. This isn't a tradition I've encountered before. It must be a Scottish thing. I don't even know what she is collecting for.

I look up. A seagull floats onto George IV's shoulder, opens its wings in a flurry, then settles.

I'll begin with Reginald D. Hunter. Years back I downloaded one of his shows.[66] Hunter is an African American man in his forties from Georgia, USA. He has made his name in the UK and is unknown in the US, a stranger in his own lands. His material covers his experience of racism both in the UK and at home, sexual etiquette and families. Each time I listen, I laugh at the familiar stories, look forward to their arrival, enjoying the craft of the writing, the way he loops back and between, the repetition of phrases and themes that appear and re-appear; how he says the unsayable, the intimate; and how, as do I, he writes about his father.

Hunter's dad is ninety-two and "his best friend in the world". The final story of the show returns to him:

They were driving together not long back. Hunter, at the wheel, says,

"Can I ask you a question?"

"Yes, anything. I've known you since you were born. Ask me anything you want, son. Anything. If you can conceive of the question, you can handle the answer".

Hunter pauses in the telling:

"You ever had anal sex?"

His dad—after Hunter has, on request, defined his terms—says no, he hasn't ever really thought about doing that; it doesn't mean anything to him. "Does it to you, son?"

"Yes", replies his son, "I have a modest appreciation".

"Ah, that's ok; everyone has their thing", says his dad, giving examples of what these might be, conveying a message of acceptance, inclusiveness, reassurance.

"Yes, everyone has their thing", his father repeats. Then adds:

"I have let a few men suck my dick though. For money".

His dad's explanation, told with offhand nonchalance, is a story of 1940s racist exploitation. The proceeds helped pay for the family's first car.

After further revelations, Hunter pulls up, gets out, sits on a bench, and takes out a joint. He instinctively thinks, "Better not. Dad won't like it" then stops, laughs and says to himself, "Fuck him. I think you'll find I don't need his approval the rest of this life".

His dad exits the car and walks over.

"You ok?"

Hunter replies, "I tell people you're my best friend in the world. How come you never told me this before?"

"Well, boy, believe me, there never was the perfect moment".

They stand to go. Hunter says,

"Wait. Wait. Is there any more?"

His dad replies,

"Oh, son, there's always more".

There's always more, always excess: in the intensities of this exchange and the implicit love and trust invoked; the transgressions we are called to believe; the shock of the mundane extraordinary; the encounter's gendered, racialized, sexualized narratives. Nothing ever exhausted or exhaustive. Always more. More humour, more sadness, more rage. In between the personal and the cultural, the intimate and the political, the ethical and less than ethical, the therapeutic or otherwise: in the telling and witnessing of stories.

The late Michael Hemmingson, in advocating stand-up as a form of, or contributor to, autoethnography, writes that he is not alone in "calling for a lighter side to autoethnography".[67] Maybe he isn't, but his comments miss the point: some stand-up works because it isn't light.

I saw Hunter live a couple of years back, in a bleak concrete theatre in the south of England. The place was full but felt cold. Hunter himself seemed flat. He hinted he'd been ill, depressed and his set was repetitive and lacked conviction. I left feeling sad and doubtful.

The hen party has long since disappeared down George Street, still no doubt calling on the unsuspecting, and I wonder. There's always more.

THERAPY: KARL

This is room four, with the chairs facing each other, the table, the clock, the window. We have done the corridor walk, silently. When I went to collect him for this, our first session, I knew who he was as the only man. Dapper, in a crisp suit and sharp tie; business attire, which is unusual. My age, perhaps; I felt under-dressed. I smiled to invite him to follow. "We're down the end", I said as he came up the couple of steps from the waiting area. I walked ahead, looking back once.

Now we sit. Karl tells me he wants therapy because he feels on the rack.

At one end the love for his wife ("Michelle, but she's always 'Shell'") and kids is grasping him by the feet, holding him to the ground. Home, stability, familiarity, responsibility. At the other, clasping his wrists, is his restlessness; pulling him, tearing at his sockets, taking him way over his head. The opposing forces have been ratcheting up these past months, imperceptible to most others, the cogs turning to tighten the pull on his core.

He isn't young for this. It's hit him later than you'd expect. Love, marriage, kids; and now the gradual, relentless, increasing tension. He feels resentful that he's got to this age, when he should be coasting towards comfort and ease and instead everything is in question.

He feels it where it hurts, in his desire. Nothing matters, nothing feels worth getting up for; and nothing feels worth getting *up* for. That would be easier to bear, if there was the usual someone else, the sly, furtive, desperate shag after a work party or the overwhelming crush and burn of a new love. At least there would be something.

So, at a comedy show the other night, he says, flanked by his wife on one side and his eldest on the other, when Katherine Ryan asked the audience if anyone had been cheated on he'd wanted to raise his hand but hadn't.

STAND-UP: KATHERINE RYAN

A Saturday evening in early August in Edinburgh. We're towards the back of an overcrowded room, in linked chairs and tight rows. We take it in turns to breathe.

August is a month of festivals in the city: highbrow international, book, art and The Fringe: comedy, music, spoken word, dance, drama, circus. Everywhere—warehouses, pubs, living rooms, pop-ups, gardens, hotels, the street—is a venue. In my building at the university, tiny classrooms, complete with dented plaster, whiteboard and mismatched tables, in a few of which I have sighed through committee meetings, become unrecognizable in black drapes, stacked seating, a PA system, lights and a stage.

The city becomes a carnival, a flood of noise and movement, colour, energy and exasperation.[68] Not everyone welcomes what the city becomes. We curse the congested pavements and the insistent, bright-eyed performers who thrust their flyers into our hands. And on each early-morning haul up the hill to work I step with disdain over the detritus of the night before.

In the centre of a row I struggle to take off my coat with dignity. We settle. The lights dim. A small blonde, curly haired cherub comes on stage, stretching her chin to the mic. She must be five or six. She tells a joke, loses her way, looks briefly off stage for help and keeps going. We think she's cute and funny and worry about her. She finishes. We laugh and cheer but don't know why she's there.

"Please welcome to the stage", she calls, "my mum, Katherine Ryan!" So we do and the girl leaves. Ryan senior touches her daughter as they pass, the little girl heading through the door and leaving us with her mum. Ryan informs us, "That was my flatmate. Did you like her?" before reassuring us that her daughter is now in the care of granny. We leave child exploitation to another day and relax.

Ryan's *shtick* is young feisty Canadian-in-Britain straight feminist. She's sharp and smart, mixing narratives of her recent life with critiques of celebrity culture, of which, of course, she is a part.

Early in the gig she tells the story of a recent "very, very, very, very, very . . ."—*Pause. Hold. Hold. Hold*—"early abortion"; of how she advised the clinic staff that she'd like to bring her flatmate—her daughter—with her, to which clinic staff frowned their disapproval. She reports how she was so well looked after she'd be happy to return; if they had wanted to put people off coming again, they should address that.

Ryan is a fan of Beyoncé, who she casts as a kick-ass, sexy, strong woman who can handle herself. Ryan does an impression of the twerking singer, together with 'don't-mess-with-me' facial expression. We admire and we laugh. We think Ryan herself must be something like this.

She discloses to the audience, "I was cheated on. Has anyone else been cheated on?" A man at the front puts up his hand. She invites him to tell his story—coming home to find his wife in bed with his friend—before she tells hers. A photo on her partner's phone, she calls the woman, who maintains it was "all right, nothing happened; it was just photos". Ryan adopts an unflattering accent to impersonate the other woman, who does not come off well in this story.

Writing

I have my feet up on the sofa in our tenement flat's back room, overlooking the courtyards and gardens of our myriad neighbours.

I am thinking about my mother, many miles south. She is often here, in a sense, though uneasily just now, as I revisit the move she has made: how it seemed as if she woke up one morning, decided she was selling her house, and within forty-eight hours had secured herself a room in a place that would accommodate her and the dog and cost thousands a month. I admire her decisiveness, love her for her boldness. Is this what T.S. Eliot meant about how as we grow old we should become explorers?[69]

Eliot's exhortation was maybe to himself. He'd just turned fifty when he started writing East Coker and he'd long since lost both parents. Anyway, he should have mentioned the cost of later life adventure. For months my siblings and I were frantic and fractious and bereft attempting to handle the financial and emotional fallout of Mum's decision and the home's neglect of due diligence.

I look outside. The leaves are fading. One low-lying tree in a courtyard in the near-distance was, for two weeks, act-of-god flame red. Now it's waning, its lustre gone.

I wonder about Katherine Ryan and loss: the sadness—integral but out of earshot—that accompanied the laughter; a hidden presence that made the laughter meaningful. The story of her abortion; those moments when she said the words; the long, long pause leading up to them. Like she knew she was somehow breaching a tacit cultural agreement, a) not to confess to an abortion, b) definitely not to do so at a stand-up gig, c) not to declare her wish that her small child—who we felt we knew and already felt protective of—accompany her and d) not to speak of having enjoyed her stay in the clinic. We went with her, though, through that story and beyond, as if there were forces in the room that took us somewhere we hadn't predicted, that took us by surprise. Something around and between and within the bodies, the tiny stage, the fibre of the red mock-plush carpet and the becoming-sweltering crowded cramp of the room. There, then gone; past; taken over by laughter, admiration, relief, Ryan's engaging irony winning us and drawing us into her narratives.

And the forces are surely different every evening. Ryan must rehearse and rehearse, repeat and repeat, script word-perfect; yet each time it must be different, each moment unique, like the moments of that Saturday evening, the affects a particular texture, and differently configured, in the confluence of there and then; she, we, we all, finding ourselves where we hadn't imagined we'd be.

Like when I speak with Mum in her new home—officially, 'Sunrise', but we call it Sunset—and she reports on her victory in the carpet putting competition, a story I have heard before—she's word-perfect—and meanwhile I have to tell her of our latest stumble in trying to secure her future there. I am pulled into love and delight and despair. Someplace I didn't exactly intend to go.[70]

And like with Karl, the man in my consulting room, where we turn and return to the tearing at his heart; and together we see if he can find a way to live with the intensities enveloping us both.

Stand-Up: Holly Walsh

Another Saturday evening in August, in a converted university seminar room, below ground, one of five off a social area with a bar and seating. The place is heaving. We queue again. It's hot again. It's a squeeze to find two seats together. We end up in the front row. We suspect we may be at risk.

Holly Walsh's show is entitled 'Never Had It'. Her hook is she doesn't have, has never had, that quality we call 'it'. She runs through a series of slides with photographs of famous faces, consulting the audience each time. Has Obama got it? Yes, we call. The Fonz? Yes. Prince Charles? No, laughing. Beyoncé yes, but not Madonna, not these days, though she did once. The audience is divided when it comes to Gary Barlow.

Walsh shows pictures of her younger self: she never had it, she argues. She was never one of the popular set at school. Those who have 'it' convey cool, whereas Walsh is a knot of uncertainty and doubt. She's ordinary, English, middle class, slight, in her 30s, recently married, drinks real ale, loves Alicia Keys and, as she tells us, looks like a younger Mary Berry.[71] She has short, blonde hair and wears blue denims and a T-shirt. She says she has only one dress. As a younger woman she was never one to drink much and her adventures into wine always ended up with her imploring "why don't you just dump me?"

We forget, or set aside, our awareness that this is a woman who is on our TV screens most weeks for some panel show or another, credible and insouciant and holding her own with the comedy boys.[72] Of course she has it, whatever she says. Yet we believe her too. Her regular everydayness is plausible and endearing.

Her set is self-deprecating and mostly about sex. Inadequate, embarrassing, failed sex. Mundane sex. Or not quite sex. Or nowhere near sex. Like the one piece of advice her mother gave her: put a towel underneath.

Walsh looks at us, at Tess and me. We thought this might happen. Walsh asks us if we're together and how long. And whether we remember the moment we first met. We struggle to answer, looking at each other, and say no but we remember the evening; it's just the moment we can't locate. She moves on: "was it love at first sight?" We look at each other again. "No", I say, "but it was like at first sight". Walsh finds this amusing.

She studied mediaeval art at Cambridge. Her particular interest was marginalia, the scribbles, comments and illuminations in the margins of ancient books. She shows us a slide of an ancient text: monks and nuns behaving spiritually and respectfully in the main picture; off the page, off stage, there's a monk with a fart trumpet, another with a finger up his rectum, and a penis tree—all sketched, she suggests, by mischievous, rebellious monks and nuns, primed by deprivation.

She compares these images to the teenage girls' magazines she grew up with and their 'sex positions of the month', sketched—showing us a slide—like her mediaeval marginalia, at the edges of the page.

THERAPY: KARL

He rubs his hands together in the cold. The heating is on but only just. The room will warm in time. I'm tired, not sleeping well. I wake in the night and am alert. I listen to the radio. Voices soothe, sometimes.

He speaks of home. He hauls himself out of bed, wakes up the children, makes coffee. Returns to hassle the reluctant ones. We're all reluctant, he says. All dragging ourselves, step by step, away from each other and towards nowhere in particular. He takes coffee to his wife in bed, the bed they no longer share. He shaves and showers. He turns on the radio, too quiet to hear above the shower or it's too loud for her. But it's muffled company, and, when the shower is off, he hears of others' bleak lives, which is a kind of comfort.

As I sit with him, I wonder what his longings are, what this tale of the sad mundane reveals and conceals. What's hiding in the margins, just off the page, in all its danger and absurdity.

STAND-UP: LUCY BEAUMONT

Lucy Beaumont is from Hull, an isolated and oft-mocked city on the east coast of England. Her gig is in a prefab on a car park next to the university gym. Getting tickets to see her has been tricky—her show has caught a mood during the month.

She is from Hull and now lives in Surrey in the comfortable southeast, but this re-location is probably temporary. She's tried to leave Hull four times. Being from Hull forms one of two related hooks for the show. The other hook is her stories of her mission to help her friend Jackie find a man. Jackie can't find a man because of Hull.

She talks as if she assumes that none of us is from or has ever been to Hull, which is probably true. Situated on an estuary in the east of the country, it's awkward to get to and isn't on the way to somewhere else. So she provides us with an induction into Hull-ness, which, for example, comes in the form of the gaudy menus she holds up from the burger bars and kebab shops down her road. She reads out the advert on each of them for the number of the NHS Helpline.

She instructs the audience to call out "Mamma Mia! Mamma Mia!" in order, we realize, to practise Hull-ese. She conducts us as we do so. In Hull, 'Mamma Mia' is telling your mother that you're home.

Beaumont performs the northern English ingénue, clutching her handbag, surrounded by pink, and telling us about holidaying in Blackpool.

Everything is a puzzle to her. She wonders why exotic foods are named as they are. She hypothesizes that they're named after the waiter or waitress that carried the original dish, the very first time it was made, to the very first table. The innovative chef creates a new recipe and, once realized and ready to carry to those who have the honour of being the first to taste it, chef shouts, "Steak, Diane!" or "Quiche, Lorraine!", or "Eggs, Benedict!", or "Eggs, Florentine!" You get the picture. "Rogan, Josh!"

The title of her show is 'We Can Twerk It Out'. Unlike Ryan's gig, here's no sign of a twerk. Despite the elusive romance theme, there's very little sex. Watching her act, twerking seems unimaginable, as far from Miley Cyrus as Surrey is from Hull.

The four of us were late in so we are split up; Tess and I are at the front, daughter Holly and friend Sam at the back. Beaumont interrupts her act—though, of course, this interruption is the act—to ask Tess to tell her the most exciting thing she has done for me. Two seconds' pause. Before Tess can answer, Holly cries out from behind us, "No, please don't". The audience laughs; I tell Beaumont unnecessarily that the voice was our daughter's.

At the end of the show, when I 'correctly' answer a question she poses (whatever answer I give would have been right), I win friend Jackie as a bride-prize, or Jackie wins me. It's not clear. Beaumont invites me up to pose for a wedding snap with a cardboard Jackie, my head through a cut-out hole, modelling like so many English holiday seaside promenade laughs. Beaumont reveals the scene to the audience, sweeping off the sheet covering the frame only when I am in place. I never see what the audience sees and finds so hilarious but imagine 'Jackie' to be bearded and me to be wearing the requisite white flowing outfit. Beaumont takes a Polaroid snap and the image begins to appear. The show ends and as we walk out there are a dozen polaroid snaps displayed on a cork board, unwitting men grinning and unsure.

THERAPY: KARL

I ask him to tell me the story of meeting his wife. He can remember the evening, he says; when it was, who they were with, that it was a show—a play, Michael Frayn—and what they talked about when they happened to be standing with drinks during the interval. He remembers it well. He remembers liking her, and knowing he wanted to see her again. He remembers the lurch in his belly that he recognized but hadn't felt for a long, long time.

There's the trace of a smile as he remembers his clumsiness at the end of the evening. He contrived to find himself walking next to her for those minutes before everyone went their own way. He knew. She knew. The others knew.

His smile is a gentle self-mocking. Affectionate. A hint; a hope.

WRITING

I caught the early morning flight south from Edinburgh and picked up a car. I stop on the motorway on the way to Mum. I buy a bottle of water, take one of the few empty tables, and read through what I've written here.

Therapy, stand-up and writing; my client, the performers, and this text.

Karl and me; and our attendance at Ryan's gig. We wonder, perhaps, about what's 'true'. What the connections are. If we were there the same night. If he is me. Client or therapist or both. Or not. In which case we wonder with whose authority I write, whose purposes I serve. Some might suggest that if stories are 'true' then their subjects are at risk, and if they aren't then the stories are hollow, just fiction.[73]

Who, what, can be believed? What about Ryan, Walsh and Hunter themselves? Was that Ryan's small child, that diminutive figure on the stage? Did Ryan have a termination? Was she cheated on? Did Walsh's mum tell her about the towel? Did Hunter's dad respond like that? Is there a dad? Did these performers tell these stories? Have I, in relaying them here, told them 'faithfully' (whatever that might mean)? Are they their stories or mine? Are those my clients' stories or my own? What has been left out? Much, of course. In all of this. It's inevitable. There's always more.

Reginald D. Hunter complains that people get offended by him. How can people be offended, he asks? Why come to a comedy gig and be offended? Don't they get they're at a *comedy* gig and therefore the guy might be joking? No, I don't buy that. The comedy works because we find a truth in it. We hold on, in faith, or we stop reading or stop listening or stop talking. Disengage. We have to keep believing or we become uncoupled. That's why we laugh, or are moved, or are offended. We stay because there's enough, just enough. We keep believing because we know 'truth' is never exact, never a simple equation of what we think of as 'experience' and the words we choose to tell of that experience; that's a story we stopped believing long ago. Truth is sly and slippery and elusive and we know this.

The issue is never whether or not stories in therapy, stand-up and writing-as-inquiry are 'true' but how they allow us in and how they come to matter. How their stories, their tellings and re-tellings, their moments and pauses, their indeterminacy and their excess, come to have weight. How they teach us. Take us. Take us with them. Take us over, overwhelming and never sufficient.

Motorway service stations become overwhelming after a time. I head to the hired car. After the short drive to Sunset, I walk through the front door of the home where two receptionists hover behind a desk in the foyer. Either side, residents sit in armchairs or wheelchairs, in clusters or alone. Some talk but most don't.

I haven't seen Mum for eight weeks. Too long. There's what they call the 'bistro' to the left where they're serving sherry before lunch. Mum is there and she introduces me to her friends. Her terrier, Mickey, circulates, restless and curious, permitting cursory petting before moving on to the next person. Most faces crease into smiles at him; some don't notice or don't care. Each time I phone or visit she tells me how popular Mickey is and I picture him leading them in group singing and hatching plots to escape.

I pull up a chair next to Mum and lean to kiss her.

"You getting drunk again?" I ask.

"Don't be silly", she replies, delighted. Mickey returns to her, jumps and settles on her lap. I'm hurting as I watch, pain resting in the margins: she is happy, and I worry she cannot stay.

NOTES

63 Richardson, *Fields of Play*, 1997. This connection between the personal and the cultural is also a claim of 'autoethnography'. Autoethnographic texts show "people in the process of figuring out what to do, how to live, and the meaning of

their struggles" (Bochner and Ellis, "Communication as Autoethnography", 2006, 111). For accounts and discussions of autoethnography, see, for example: Adams, Holman Jones, and Ellis, *Autoethnography*, 2014; Ellis, *The Ethnographic I*, 2004, *Revision*, 2009); Ellis, Adams, and Bochner, "Autoethnography: An Overview", 2011; Short, Turner, and Grant, *Contemporary British Autoethnography* 2013. There are many other good sources. Although there are connections between autoethnography and writing-as-inquiry, it is writing-as-inquiry that I work with in this book because of its congruence with the book's theoretical framings.

64 See Spry, *Body, Paper, Stage*, 2011.

65 More often with women stand-up performers than men. See Gilbert, *Performing Marginality*, 2004.

66 Hunter, "Reginald D. Hunter Live", 2011.

67 Hemmingson, "Make Them Giggle", 2008, 10.

68 Like Pelias' Bourbon Street: "beyond the everyday, an enticing place that bewitches and beguiles". Pelias, "A Personal History of Lust on Bourbon Street", 2006, 56.

69 Eliot, *Four Quartets*, 2009.

70 I appropriate Stewart, *Ordinary Affects*, 2007, 79, here.

71 A UK celebrity chef.

72 Yes, they're still mostly boys. See Gilbert, *Performing Marginality*, 2004.

73 As Peter Clough discusses. Clough, *Narratives and Fictions in Educational Research*, 2002.

INTERVAL[74]

Towards Creative-Relational Inquiry (1): Take It to Heart

Early 2018, Edinburgh

In this chapter, the first of three 'Intervals' that spend time with 'creative-relational inquiry', I begin from Brian Massumi's use of the term, 'creative-relational', before writing into examples from and about therapy, stand-up, and writing as a method of inquiry. In doing so, I draw from those both elsewhere within the book (looking backwards and forwards) and beyond it, to help in considering the possibilities creative-relational inquiry opens up. I also propose that creative-relational inquiry calls, not for 'writing as a method of inquiry', but 'writing-as-inquiry'. In the second of these three intervals, I argue for the place of the personal in such creative-relational inquiry; in the third I consider the concept's hyphen.

In proposing *creative-relational inquiry*, I take my cue from Canadian theorist, Brian Massumi, who—in what may seem a long way from therapy, stand-up and writing, but bear with me—argues for a different understanding of evolutionary processes. He proposes how the received wisdom of understanding evolution as pure (and only) adaptation is inadequate and leaves unacknowledged the degree of improvisation required; and by improvisation he means:

> a modification rising from *within* an activity's stirring, bringing a qualitative difference to its manner of unfolding. It is immanent to the activity's taking its own course.[75]

In other words, the something new that happens takes place in the act, in the process. Instead of the concept of adaptation, Massumi continues, it is much more convincing to speak in terms of Deleuze and Guattari's *becoming*, or emergence: a becoming pulled "deformationally, creatively ahead, outside common sense",[76] pulled—and, surely, pushed—in particular by desire, "a force of liaison, a force of linkage, conveying a transformational tendency".[77]

This desire takes the animal's becoming towards the 'supernormal' of "life's exceeding itself".[78] Massumi writes:

> Take it to heart: animal becoming is *most* human. It is in becoming animal that the human recurs to what is nonhuman at the heart of what moves it. This makes its surpassingly human. Creative-relationally *more-than* human.[79]

The creative-relational, for Massumi, is therefore what characterizes a process of becoming that takes it, the animal, the human, us, beyond ourselves, into the other, into becoming-other, into the more-than. Desire is the push and pull, the draw, the force of the creative-relational; the force that connects, the force that leans us towards (the) other, towards becoming-other, towards movement, towards change. Desire is the creative-relational gesture that means we can't not go beyond ourselves, can't not spill out, can't not become caught up in the im/possibility[80] of life's excess.

Take it to heart, writing as a method of inquiry is creative-relational. Writing as a method of inquiry reaches out beyond us, reaches in to where we may not want to go, a 'minor gesture'[81] towards that which we do not know, to that which is beyond us:

> There's something about writing books that is out of time. As though the writing only really knows what it's after once it has begun to make its way into the world. For me, thinking too has always had this quality: thinking thickens in its encounter with the futurity that orients it. This futurity in thinking's presentness is part of what keeps thinking lithe: thinking is always out of sync with itself. The best kind of encounter with thinking's outside is the kind that deeply listens to what writing is trying to do, almost thinking beyond what the author is capable of thinking, then returning that thinking, almost beyond what the reader can think, to the author. In

this gesture of encounter, no one is trying to convince anyone: thought is thinking collectively at its limit.[82]

Writing is thinking:[83] writing-thinking. Writing-thinking is lithe, writing-thinking is an encounter.[84] It is writing-as-creative-relational-inquiry; and it is writing-as-inquiry, not writing as a *method of* inquiry.[85] 'Method' belongs to the procedural, to the linear and the sequential, the reified and the stratified of 'research methods'. Writing-as-inquiry, Jackson might say, is "thinking without method".[86] Writing-as-inquiry is process, creative-relational in its various fluid, dynamic, forceful, hyphenated encounters: writer-reader, beyond-writer-beyond-reader-beyond; book-world-time; writing-thinking-outside-listening; present-future; and (in no particular order) writing-thinking-future-present.[87]

***

Pause. Those three stars there, the *dinkus*,[88] forming the line above, indicate as much, giving me permission. A chance to look up, look out. Look around—9.41am, 9 January 2018—months, years, later than many sections of this book, the sequencing ragged, or as if ragged; as if any book is written as it appears to be, one word after another. The present-past-future-ness of writing.

It seems dark outside still. It *is* dark outside still, but it feels like it shouldn't be at this time of the morning so I'm trying to persuade myself. Yet it's winter (again) and from my desk I can see there's a swathe of dull cloud beyond the window, above the bare trees and church tower.

Soon I will be interrupted (let's say intra-rupted, a rupture arising from an ontological *within*) by Alan who has re-painted our main room while we were travelling over the Christmas and New Year break. He's coming around to check we're happy with his work and to collect payment. He wants cash (please don't tell) and my desk drawer is stuffed full of notes. I like him. I hope he arrives soon. He likes to talk so the intra-ruption might be longer than you imagine and longer than I feel I deserve.

I need him to arrive so I can take a break from this. Am I making too much of writing? It's a question I keep asking. It's a question born of both frustration and curiosity. My frustration (and my curiosity) is how I return to this point, this precise point, in the text, trying to make it work. Trying to connect with it. Trying to *make sense* of it. Not an 'easy sense' but a sense that lives and works with the complexities, contradictions and silences.[89] A sense that *feels* its way into it, touching it, and touching beyond it, outside, reaching, in order to be open to the possibility of thinking otherwise.[90] How can I be with it, encounter it, so it/I can come alive? At this point I can't (or feel I can't) so I want to push it away, push writing's claims away, push Manning away, push away from—rather than reach towards—an argument for the creative-relational of writing.

Maybe I'm trying too hard to *know*, trying too hard to be smart. Maybe I need to allow myself to become a *dinkus*.

'Writing-as-inquiry' sounds so open-ended, so inviting, so free. See where it goes, it calls, see what writing opens up; trust it, allow it to take you where it wills. I issue students with such invitations but at this moment, here, waiting for Alan to arrive, "[writing stalls] in its encounter with the futurity that orients it"[91] as the deadline for completing this book—less than seven months and it's already been years in the writing—comes into view. The future is now, folded into this moment, as I seem only to sit, write and delete. Write, delete. Write, delete, in snatched early morning moments gazing at the screen before the world awakes.

Perhaps, under pressure, I lose faith in what else writing is, other than writing. Novelist Jon McGregor writes how he is often asked the time it takes to write a novel. It depends upon what they mean, he says:

> [T]he work that actually happens at a desk is not always time spent actually writing. There are other things that happen. There are other sorts of time, besides writing time. There is thinking time, reading time, research time and sketching out ideas time. There is working on the first page over and over again until you find the tone you're looking for time. There is spending just five minutes catching up on email time. There is spending five minutes more on Twitter, because, in a way, that is part of the research process time. There is writing time, somewhere in there.[92]

Yes, I forget, lose faith, that reading is also writing, even at this point, the deadline in view, when the word count at the foot of the page is what matters most. I lose faith that it is important to think—and to allow writing to think, to allow writing to think towards what I am unable to imagine.

Writing stalls in the shadow of a publisher's deadline. Writing stalls also in its encounter with mortality: my mother's deterioration over the past year, since her January 2016 fall rendered her using a wheelchair and without use of her right arm. I want to—have to—be able to sit alongside her, with Mickey on her lap, holding a manuscript in my hand, saying, "here, I have something for you". To which she will reply, "Oh, thank you. But what is it? What's it about?", and then, "Have you written about me? There's not much to write about me, though, is there? Not like there was with Dad". To which I will say, "Yes, you're in it and there was plenty to say. Shall I read it to you?", leaving unanswered her question of what the book is about.

I must write, whatever writing is and whatever its claims. There isn't much time. And I want to write. There is curiosity. There is desire.

Take it to heart.

***

Take it to heart.

Massumi suggests the creative-relational is a process of becoming, with desire as its force. Creative-relational *inquiry*, then, may be conceptualized as inquiry that seeks not to 'capture' and hold still, but to find a way, through desire, to do justice to the fluidity of process. Creative-relational inquiry takes up not (only) the common-sense understanding of creative—notions of making, of 'being artistic', etc.—but the radical, creative opening-up-to-what-may-be, an opening-up within "an encounter [that] is not a confrontation with a 'thing' but a *relation* that is sensed, rather than understood".[93] Creativity as *becoming*.[94] As Ken Gale and I write,

> Creative practices of concept forming, always involving active conceptualisation, are the very processual activities that trouble the reified substantialities of conventional inquiry. They are not simply about changing the concept from one thing, one classified object of inquiry, to another through practices of critical interpretation, they involve selves in doing, in engaging in affective forms of inquiry that animate doing-bodies in ethical, political and always experimentally-infused ways.[95]

Creative-relational inquiry is about movement, about process. The creative-relational keeps us guessing, is marked by its unfolding, by the promise of the not-yet, by unpredictability.

Creativity as process, relating as process.

Like[96] how, in therapy, when Karl tells me about first meeting his wife, the story of that sensing-memory of a brush of shoulders and its (al)chemical release, something is conjured in that moment between us. Something more than us, something outside inside, inside outside; and something gone, then there. Something we might call hope.

Like, again in therapy, when Karl and I come to know that without the two of us being in that room together—though we have always been more than two—at that moment, and each week over the past many months, we never would have understood how rare, how precious, this encounter has been in his becoming aware that he matters, both to himself and to me.

Therapy: creative-relational inquiry.

And like, in stand-up, how Reginald D. Hunter brings his father to us. We share a car journey with them. He summons their world. He takes us into their intimacy.

Like how, last summer,[97] in a marquee in George Square Gardens, Sarah Kendall performed the intricate intertwining family stories of her stand-up show, *One Seventeen*.[98] She swept us between the years of her lives in an inquiry into luck, loving and loss as she told of gazing at the stars with her father, of living with her autistic son and being abducted by aliens. Prompted by a member of the audience, at one point she executed a spontaneous cartwheel across the stage that took us spinning with her into possible worlds. Now you see her, now you don't.

Like how, in the Adam GC Riches show that same month, as he cast the two members of the audience he'd 'invited' from the front row—their resistance futile—in the scene of a couple declaring and writing love to each other, the movement of bodies, the laughter, the imagination, the energy, the surprise, all caught us in its magic and we became what we weren't.[99] Believing, hoping, trusting, aghast, in the semi-circle of tiered seats watching the young woman dictating her declaration of love while her 'lover' wrote her words in mock-blood, blindfolded, onto the performer's T shirt. You had to be there. We went with it, finding ourselves otherwise in the absurdity of the burgeoning moment.

Stand-up: creative-relational inquiry.

And like how, with writing, a sense of longing and loss can find a way into form as my mother raises her glass of sherry to me one Sunday lunchtime.

Like how, again with writing and with loss, I might find a way to write into how loss changes, shifts, is never still: our adult son's sudden near-fatal road accident on the other side of the world[100] and the jolt into life's precariousness; those hours of uncertainty as we wait to hear news; the surges of shock and disbelief; then after many days, relief. And how, a year, two years, three years on, it's still there, that mark on the calendar, that mark on our bodies, a continuing unfolding as he, we, all, continue to become something other than we were.

Writing: creative-relational inquiry.

***

Take it to heart. Inquiry such as this renders therapist, performer and writer in motion too: affected, involved, implicated, never able to be distant and separate, always caught up, caught up in the flow, only ever able to seek a way to shape that which is partial, momentary, always already transforming.

Creative-relational inquiry sees the process of relating itself as creative. Creative-relational inquiry casts relating—to others, to ourselves, to the material world—as generative process, as doing, as dynamic. Creative-relational inquiry hints at the possible in relating. How 'we', bodies, meaning, life, are created in and through relating. The creative-relational acknowledges how *relata*—we, me, you, this—are produced through the relational.[101] The process of relating comes first.

Like how this wooden table, with my left hand, my writing hand, leaning on the black-covered notebook decorated in the red mandala sketch drawn for me, a gift, my right forearm taking the weight of my leaning torso, the black bookmark cast up and back, the teacups for our guests—asleep downstairs—resting at the table's centre, the pale wooden chair on which I sit, the early morning bustle outside as the city awakes, and more, are in relation, in touch, and this relating is creating this, us, me.

Such a take on relating hints, obliquely, at how de Freitas, drawing upon Karen Barad, speaks of the "queer alteration of relationality".[102] Not a humanist, anthropocentric relationality that blandly claims 'everything is connected', but a quantum relationality where:

> Touch becomes the fundamental relation of the world—a quivering quantum tug that holds us together, rather than a classical physical collision

encounter. [Karen Barad] claims that this quantum touch stretches across the inhuman field of virtual indeterminacy and can furnish an ethics adequate to the world.[103]

Touch in this framing is more than what we commonly understand—skin on skin—though it would include this too. Touch is the push/pull of relating that makes us—relating across time, across substances, across species. Touch is a "gesture of exchange with the world", writes walker/writer Robert MacFarlane in *The Old Ways*, his book on ancient pathways: "[T]he soles of our feet, shaped by the surfaces they press upon, are landscapes themselves with their own worn channels and roving lines".[104] For de Freitas, for Barad, touching is what language *does*: "language is a kind of haptic/touch relation that *inheres* in the world and perhaps *expresses* the world".[105] How writing touches.[106]

***

Until now this has been the same as every other week:

The walk from the waiting area along the corridor, dog-legging left to room 4, me slightly ahead of Karl, the two of us silent.

I had ducked my head, as always, under one of the ceiling lights, just that one and none of the others and only on the way to the room. I never need to. I know this. It must be something about the angle of approach, the way I see it from that direction that means I view it as a risk, and a risk I must not take.

I had pushed the door and held it open for him, as always, closing it behind as he passed me and walked past my chair.

He had shed his coat and bag and flopped onto his chair, having first removed from it the blue cushion he never wants to use. Once, many weeks ago, I remembered before he arrived and placed it on the floor, but I have never remembered since.

I, as always, had taken my own seat and shuffled it back a few inches to give us more space. I forget before he arrives the two of us like to stretch out our legs, which can feel too intimate.

Until now it has been like this, just the same:

He has caught me up on his week, told me about continued stresses at work, told me how tired he is, told me how nothing has changed at home.

I have sat still, mostly, noticing my struggle to stay with him. Occasionally, I have shifted position to being cross-legged on the chair, which I like to do. It stretches me, aligns me, helps me be more aware of the activity, the sense, of my body, more able to be present.

However, I have been leaving the room. I have been taken to the pressing tasks I must get done by tomorrow. I have been taken to Mum and how I forgot—again—to call her this morning. 11.00am is the best time to call because she's always in the lounge for coffee and the staff can take the phone to her, but I am always caught up in other matters and am not thinking about her.

I have not felt in touch. Not with here, this room, this evening. Not with my sense of myself, nor with Karl, however I have sat, and however I have attempted to pay attention to what's happening. Something is happening, I know that, but I'm nowhere near it. There feels a stasis in him, in me, in us. I look at him. I try to look at him, differently, so as to hear him/us, leaning to rest my head on the fingers of my right hand, my right elbow on the arm of the chair.

He has not spoken for maybe a minute. It feels a long time.

"What is it you want from me?", he asks.

"Tonight, you mean? Now? Or generally, from this?"

"Now".

Everything has changed. That question, arising, erupting, and I am alert, here, present. His tone is curious, like he's wanting to work out the rules of this game. It's a challenge, but I don't hear it as angry, which it might have been. He looks at me. Just then, it is like we have never met. I am shocked.

The usual responses won't do. I can't push it back to him. I can't offer the stock therapist response, though they're what come to me immediately to me; questions like, "What do you imagine I want?" or "What is it you want from you?"

What do I want from him? To entertain me? Or to not keep doing everything we always do? To help us find a break in the current, slow, metre of our encounter, opening us to rhythm?[107] Am I waiting for him to fall so I can rescue him? For him to dislodge a divot as he slips on the smooth grass, which, like Shannon, Sedgwick's therapist, I would pick up and replace?[108]

"What do you want from me?", he repeats, sadder now in my silence, as I fail to respond.

What do I want from him? What do I want from him? I hear the question echo and look away, as he has done too. No longer the challenge in his eyes, nor in the tone of his voice.

"I can't find an answer to what you've asked me. I've been trying to, but nothing seems to fit".

We're back looking at each other, for a moment, then away again. I've shifted in my seat again and I sense something shift in us. He's still. I can hear an ambulance siren pass, some way off. The room is sheltered, at the rear of the building.

"What do I want from you. . . ." I find myself saying, not knowing where I'm going. "I want you to. . . . I want us to . . . keep trying. . . ." I tail off. Then, "That's all I've got. Keep trying".

"Like Sisyphus".

"Like Sisyphus, yes".

"You know, keep heaving the load up the mountain, only we'll never reach the top. The load will always be too much and we'll start over again at the bottom. Over and over".

"I see".

"Keep trying, because that's all we can do. Sisyphus. You know your Greek myths?"

Then adds,

"Only it's me, not 'we'. It's my load, not ours, isn't it?"

"Yet, perhaps, there is the possibility here of the load not staying the same, exactly as it has always been. It can change shape, it can change size".

He seems to let this find its way. He looks up. I say,

"And we can, at least during this time, hold it together".

***

The creative-relational inquiry of therapy—and stand-up, and writing—works at and with the routines of the ordinary and the everyday,[109] with the struggle of the uneasy, of not being able to find a way, of missing each other. Creative-relational inquiry also works at and with the moments of surprise,[110] moments when something happens, something not 'mine' or 'Karl's', but something beyond technique, beyond behaviour, beyond us. Something more-than. Always more.

Take it to heart, Massumi invokes in the lines that prompt the start of this chapter and I have kept repeating. "Take it to heart". I can't let that instruction, that invitation, go. "Take it to heart". Not the romantic, humanist heart, but a heart of the more-than. Beating, rhythmic, racing, the heart that goes out, the one that does not 'belong' only to the body it beats in. It takes me to asserting: there is a 'heart' to the creative-relational, there is a heart to creative-relational inquiry. We can say there can be, even, the *personal*. A personal that is dynamic, hyphenated, late, collective, provisional; a personal in the chapters that have preceded and in those that follow, and personal I discuss further in the next 'Interval'.

NOTES

74 In a typical local stand-up show, the evening is broken up into—or 'striated' by, as Deleuze and Guattari might say—three or four segments, with a break in between, an interval, a time for replenishing glasses, talking and visiting the bathroom. But the apparent 'brokenness', the intervals, does not create 'gaps'. The intervals are not empty, they are lively and active; they feed, fold, into the performances that follow (as well as those that have preceded them). They are 'smooth spaces' where things happen. Similarly, in this book, the intervals are substantive: "There are stops and trajectories in both the smooth and the striated. But in smooth space, the stop follows from the trajectory; once again, *the interval takes all, the interval is substance*". Deleuze and Guattari, *A Thousand Plateaus*, 2004, 528, my emphasis.

75 Brian Massumi, "The Supernormal Animal", 2015, 7. My emphasis.

76 Massumi, 9.

77 Massumi, 9. Massumi's is a Deleuzian take on desire: not desire as psychoanalysis' lack but desire as productive. Rajchman elaborates: "(W)e need another picture of unconscious desire itself and the kind of 'complex' it forms that is no longer 'transgressive' or 'sacrificial'; we should rather see it in a 'constructivist' manner in terms of this informal plane through which our libidinal virtualities are played out". Rajchman, *The Deleuze Connections*, 2000, 91.

78 Massumi, "The Supernormal Animal", 2015, 14.

79 Massumi, 14. Italics in the original.

80 I am taking the use of the slash—/—from Karen Barad, to indicate not either/or (or even both/and) but a dynamic between one and the other, "an active and reiterative (intra-active) rethinking of the binary": how, in this case, possibility and impossibility are not opposite or mutually exclusive but constantly seeking out and spinning off each other. Juelskjær and Schwennesn, "Intra-Active Entanglements", 2012, 19.

81 Manning, *The Minor Gesture*, 2016. I want to connect Manning's 'minor gesture', in particular in relation to writing as taken up here by Manning and then me, with Cixous' claim for writing being a "gesture of love. *The* gesture"

(see Chapter 2). I see their 'gestures' as potentially congruent if Cixous' writing gesture of love is seen not as a transcendent but as an immanent practice, a "gestural force that opens experience to its potential variation. It does this from within experience itself, activating a shift in tone, a difference in quality". Manning, 1.

82 Manning, ix.

83 This echoes St. Pierre in Richardson and St. Pierre, "Writing: A Method of Inquiry", 2017, 827: "[W]riting *is* thinking, writing *is* analysis, writing *is* indeed a seductive and tangled *method* of discovery", emphasis in the original.

84 An encounter, for Deleuze, is "not a confrontation with a 'thing' but a *relation* that is sensed, rather than understood" (Jackson, "Thinking Without Method", 2017, 669). An encounter is "[s]omething in the world [that] forces us to think" (Deleuze, *Difference and Repetition*, 2004, 176).

85 Although, as St. Pierre argues, Richardson's use of the term 'method' in 'writing as a method of inquiry' is deconstructive, in any case, creating space for different ways to conceptualize the term. Richardson and St. Pierre, "Writing: A Method of Inquiry", 2017.

86 Jackson, "Thinking Without Method", 2017.

87 I do more work with the hyphen of creative-relational inquiry in Interval 3.

88 According to the Urban Dictionary a dinkus is also "a person that does stupid things. An insult. When you act like an idiot, you are being a Dinkus". Just saying. www.urbandictionary.com/define.php?term=Dinkus.

89 Mazzei, "Beyond An Easy Sense", 2014.

90 Jackson, "Thinking Without Method", 2017.

91 To paraphrase Manning, *The Minor Gesture*, 2016, ix.

92 McGregor, "My Working Day", 2018.

93 Jackson, "Thinking Without Method", 2017, 669, emphasis in the original.

94 Harris, *The Creative Turn*, 2014.

95 Gale and Wyatt, "Riding the Waves", 2018, 203.

96 I am drawing from Erin Manning and Brian Massumi here and at other points in the text in this deployment of 'like': 'like', here, is indicative of both particularity and excess, both proposing something specific and, at the same time, being suggestive of the 'always more': "'[L]ike' . . . marks an affective overflow in speech. This feeling is just sad. More than that, it is just like sad is. It refracts all sadness, and its difference from happiness, in the singular feeling this is". Manning and Massumi, "JUST LIKE THAT", 2016, 122.

97 August 2017.

98 At the Edinburgh Fringe, August 2017.

99 "The Inane Chicanery of a Certain Adam GC Riches", Edinburgh, August 2017.

100 See Chapter 11.

101 Barad, *Meeting the Universe Halfway*, 2007.

102 de Freitas, "Karen Barad's Quantum Ontology and Posthuman Ethics", 2017, 747.

103 de Freitas, 747.

104 MacFarlane, *The Old Ways*, 2012, 161.

105 de Freitas, "Karen Barad's Quantum Ontology and Posthuman Ethics", 2017, 747.

106 Wyatt *et al.*, "How Writing Touches", 2011; Gale *et al.*, *How Writing Touches*, 2012.

107 This is an allusion to Guattari's, and Deleuze and Guattari's, 'refrain'. See Chapters 4 and 5.

108 Sedgwick, "A Dialogue on Love", 1998. However, 'Shannon', Sedgwick's therapist, makes this gesture not knowing the piece of turf had been dislodged by Sedgwick, nor that Sedgwick happened to see him do so, "encountering my ghost without recognition, unmaking my mistake—me, turning back, seeing it. And I love that his care for me was not care for *me*". 631.

109 See Chapter 5, "The Refrains of Therapy and the Everyday".

110 See Chapter 4, "What Has Stand-up Ever Done for Writing-as-Inquiry: The Refrain, Surprise, Pete, and His Lemons".

Part 2

Refrains[111]

---

111 The first two chapters of this section of the book work with Deleuze and Guattari's concept of the 'refrain'. They do this in relation, respectively, to stand-up and writing and then (primarily) to therapy and the everyday. Refrains—or, perhaps better, the verb, the process, 'refraining'—continue(s) to run through the following three chapters. The chapters pick up, in turn, on 'shit', performing stand-up and father-son relating.

Chapter 4

WHAT HAS STAND-UP EVER DONE FOR WRITING-AS-INQUIRY? THE REFRAIN, SURPRISE, PETE, AND HIS LEMONS

January–March 2016, Edinburgh

This is the first of two linked chapters that work with Guattari's, and Deleuze and Guattari's, concept of 'the refrain'. In the first of these chapters I find myself lured into how stand-up comedy speaks to writing-as-inquiry. I follow a performance by a local comic, Pete, at The Stand's Monday evening new material night, Red Raw, into thinking about surprise and the 'refrain', and from there into the refrain and writing. In the following chapter I explore the links between the refrain and therapy.

Monday, 11 January 2016, Red Raw

I head up the hill to The Stand for tonight's Red Raw, the weekly 'beginner's showcase'. I imagine it will be less busy than the weekend shows—it's a Monday and there are no stars performing—so I saunter there after a leisurely dinner and arrive with just twenty minutes until showtime. I drop down the steps to the porch, pay my two-pound fee, and realize as I venture in that there is barely even standing room. I see a space in the frieze of bodies against the back wall, but the guy next to it says he's saving it for friends getting the drinks. Instead I squeeze into a corner by the hatch at the side of the bar. Staff come and go, moving with purpose and intent, empty glasses stacked. I expect to be moved on as a health and safety hazard but they ignore me.

The crowd is a-buzz. It's unexpected, perhaps, this sense of antici-pation. After all we know what's going to happen: the techie will give the five-minute warning, lower the lights and lead us in cheering on the MC; the MC will do the warm-up; a series of acts will do their thing either side of two intervals; end. This is the shape of live stand-up and it's familiar. Nonetheless, the room is full of hope. Something might happen.

The audience is younger than at the weekends, mostly students. I am the senior citizen here: an old guy standing in the corner by the bar on his own with a bottle of Sol, writing in a notebook. The staff have me clocked as not only in the way but suspect.

The lights dim, the opening bars of Reet Petite issue their summons and the techie roars on the MC. The MC is 'The Wee Man', a hyper-active crop- and bleach-haired Glaswegian who warms us up by entic-ing an earnest guy in the front row, Kramer, onto the stage as his good-natured, goofy stooge for an unlikely rap about a night on the town. Somehow, it works, with Kramer taking the ribbing well and the MC conveying warmth. He has won us round, and he gets Kramer to lead the wave of applause for the first act.

***

Writing about stand-up and therapy over recent years I have found myself drawn to how stand-up might act as a 'provocation'[112] for conceptualiz-ing writing-as-inquiry. In what follows I find myself thinking, first, with and about surprise, which takes me into Deleuze and Guattari's 'refrain' and from there into writing-as-inquiry and back to stand-up.

TAKEN BY SURPRISE

Reginald D. Hunter tells the story of when he was a teenager endur-ing a fractious relationship with his mother and he (I paraphrase) "got caught up in a bad crowd. I started experimenting".[113] We expect him to say, "experimenting with drugs" or perhaps a more specific substance ("experimenting with dope"?). After all, he was a teenager and that's what teenagers experiment with when they get caught up in bad crowds. We are waiting for that line: instead he says, "I got caught up in a bad crowd. I started experimenting with sarcasm".

The unexpectedness of this delights and we laugh. We form a picture of the teenager getting high on sarcasm, unable to stop using it, 'consuming' it in different forms and quantities, observing the effect it has on both himself and others. There is jeopardy present, even though we know the dangerous territory he is exploring is only words. In fact, the sense of peril is heightened because we know the context is his conflicted relationship with his mother. ("You need to know I hated my mother", he says.) We know his mother does not welcome this new development. We know there is trouble ahead, and we look forward to hearing about it.

I am coming at surprise here not from the perspective of wanting to understand it, break it down or reduce it to ordered technique, nor from a desire to explain or teach it, but in a spirit of seeking to be surprised by surprise, to be astounded at and by its *ontology*. We are 'caught' by surprise. As an audience we like that we do not see Hunter's next line coming. We like that our expectations are disrupted. We like that our clichéd understandings of adolescence are challenged. We are *caught, taken, by surprise*.

Surprise is substantively documented within the literature on humour and comedy. There is, for example, the way in which a joke can be structured first around the establishing of a narrative, then by its reinforcement, followed by its subversion.[114] For example: I had a few beers to get me through writing this chapter. (Narrative established.) Writing, as we know, is tough work. (Reinforcement.) But it would have been easier without the students there, waiting for my lecture to start. (Subversion.) This is surprise as technique, as something the performer *does*. However, I am not interested here in technique, not interested in how the comedian does it, but drawn instead to how Stewart Lee, in describing the pleasure of surprise in humour, begins to hint at how surprise *arises*:

> [There is the pleasure of] things being simply unexpected and wrong, of reversing the usual order of things. Surprise is the reason a one-year-old child laughs if you put a shoe on your head. Shoes are for feet, not heads. Even a baby has a sense of inappropriate behaviour.[115]

Although Lee focuses upon what the adult does, there is the sense of surprise and its humour being found in the space in-between, happening. This is surprise as onto-epistemological disruption,[116] surprise as an affect that picks us up and places us somewhere else; something that happens, that erupts, that grabs both adult and baby, performer and audience alike (and writer/researcher and reader), transporting us all. The flow of affect that emerges 'qualified', as Massumi puts it, as what we choose to call surprise.[117] It is 'captured', for a moment, in our bodies, before it moves on and returns to the excess whence it came. The *ontology* of surprise. It is this take on surprise that I develop further in this chapter, through Deleuze and Guattari's figure of 'the refrain', first in relation to stand-up and then in relation to writing-as-inquiry, though the linearity of this is troubling: the writing-as-inquiry is happening now as well as later in the chapter; and now, in January 2016 as well as now/later as I revisit and revise in June 2018, and at various points in between.

Monday, 11 January 2016, Red Raw

I have seen Pete perform before. I know him only as Pete and I didn't catch his surname when the Wee Man announced him over the cheering and whooping. Pete and I were on the same bill twice last year, at a time when he was finishing his PhD. On the second occasion he was the final act, the headline. Later this evening, after his performance, at the bar during the interval, he will tell me that he now has a postdoctoral position, which keeps him in Edinburgh while he works his way up the Edinburgh comedy tree. An aspiring comedian with an academic day-job to pay the bills.

He's in his thirties, shaven-headed, medium height, pleasant; ordinary perhaps. A regular guy. And on stage he's casual, like he walked out to get milk and found himself at the mic. I haven't seen him do this set before, the heart of which concerns his mental health. "I'm sad", he tells the audience, then explains that he has been to his doctor a number of times about 'feeling sad'. He refuses to take medication, and his refusal apparently frustrates the doctor. On each visit the doctor gives him the same questionnaire to complete, one question of which asks Pete if he has "considered suicide". Pete muses on this question. He objects, he tells us, to the word 'considers': "Over the past week, have you considered suicide?" it asks. This 'considers' is a sticking point. He tells us he 'considers' many things. He considers, for example, when he is standing in the fruit and veg section of the supermarket, lobbing a lemon into nearby aisles. He considers whether a grapefruit might do the job, but a grapefruit is too large. He considers a plum, but a plum is too small. But he considers a lemon and a lemon sits snug in the palm of your hand. The supermarket is a good place to lob a lemon—much better than, say, at home—because there is a good range of choices, there are people around and, with the aisles, they wouldn't know the source of the flying yellow fruit.

I am entranced by this segment of his set. We all are, I venture. We are Pete, in the fruit and veg section, weighing the possibilities along with fruit. We feel the satisfaction that comes with considering the risky and the socially prohibited. We are willing him to do it. We are in the breakfast cereals aisle three rows along watching unsuspecting shoppers who never see the lemon coming and we run away, sniggering and triumphant.

Slow and hesitant, Pete continues by saying that it is true that he 'considers' chucking lemons in the supermarket but it doesn't mean he perpetrates the act; so it may be the case that he 'considers' suicide but considering the act does not mean he will do it or will even get close to doing it. What therefore is the doctor's questionnaire trying to get at? Furthermore, he questions why the doctor persists with giving it to him each time. He wonders aloud with us: is the doctor trying to tell him something? Is the doctor perhaps suggesting that instead of trying his patience by returning repeatedly only to refuse his advice Pete should more than consider taking his own life? He should just do it and get out of his hair.

Pete ends with reassurance that we don't need to feel worried about him, that he is fine; and, anyway, it is possible he is not 'sad' at all, possible none of this has been true. It could be the case he has not been seeing a doctor for depression; that he has never considered the merits of throwing lemons in the supermarket; that he has been taking us for a ride. If he has been lying, if that is the case, he says, that would be terrible. Wrong. Shameful. Unforgivable. He lowers his head, turns and hurries off the stage. The audience is uncertain. We think we laugh. We applaud, but with only one hand; then we get it—he's gone—and we give him a more decisive send-off. But we're still not sure.

I'm not sure: I'm annoyed with him. Don't cast doubt like that, Pete. Don't call what you've been saying into question, especially about the lemons. That wasn't the deal you made with us. Bastard.

SURPRISE, THE REFRAIN AND STAND-UP

Pause. Think: about how this segment of Pete's set takes us; about what happens; about how it catches us by surprise. It is in this sense that Guattari's—Guattari, the pianist[118]—and then Deleuze and Guattari's, conceptualizing of the refrain provides a way to think about surprise in relation to Pete.

Alecia Jackson works with the refrain—Plateau 11 of *A Thousand Plateaus*—in a complex, beautiful paper, in which she offers a narrative drawn from her research encounter with a high school cheerleader.[119] The girl has "punk sensibilities",[120] is dressed not in cheerleader's uniform but in her own casual clothes, has the 'wrong'-shaped body for cheerleading's highly conformist, 'molar'[121] milieu, and when she is called upon in both rehearsal and performance to do the expected final move (lift up skirt back, rotate hips) instead performs a backflip. Jackson employs the concept of the refrain—"something that is repeated to produce rhythmic difference"[122]—to examine the emergence of the backflip.

Jackson outlines the refrain's three 'movements', as explored in Plateau 11. They are not sequential but are three angles on the refrain, all simultaneously present. First, a refrain is an act suggestive of order amongst chaos: a tentative, open gesture that gathers, for a moment, at the "threshold of disorder or degeneration", like "a child singing in the dark to ward off fear".[123] Second, a refrain stakes a claim, albeit fragile, to territory, "to establish both a dimensional and non-dimensional space of solitude and isolation",[124] such as, Jackson suggests, someone who uses head phones to establish privacy in busy places, a privacy that can be disturbed by knocking into a passer-by or by a friend tapping them on a shoulder.

The third movement of the refrain concerns how it both demarcates space and signals towards territory beyond that space. It cuts together/apart[125] and thereby opens up the possibility of something else, something different; improvisation; a line of flight:

> the demarcated space defines a territory beyond it but that is created by it, in the world or in the future. . . . [The refrain] is an invocation of the cosmos, an opening to the outside.[126]

Deleuze, in conversation with Clare Parnet, illustrates what he and Guattari mean, suggesting how one might hum while doing housework, or hum while travelling, anxious to get home, or hum when leaving home to go elsewhere. The refrain concerns territory:

> [It] is absolutely linked to the problem of territory, and of processes of entrance or exit of the territory, meaning the problem of deterritorialisation. I enter my territory, I try, or I deterritorialise myself, meaning I leave my territory.[127]

Picture Pete entering the stage, cheered on by the small, cramped crowd. He is the last performer before the interval. He has followed a guy who thought he was good but wasn't and the audience is hopeful but not confident Pete will be different. Pete stands at the mic, which he moves between leaving fixed on the stand and detaching and holding in his hand. He speaks of the questionnaire's enquiry, the questionnaire he completes visit after visit after visit. Picture how he once again enters his GP's surgery and sits in the usual chair by the desk. His GP frowns and hands him the paperwork. "Have you ever considered suicide?", the questionnaire asks; and hear how Pete is telling us this now, in this darkened basement. The "demarcated space" of that small wooden stage creates the territory of this encounter, of the question of 'considering suicide'; it is a whistling in the dark, a darkness that others in the room will know or can imagine. Hear him imagining lemons thrown into the air, over the food shelves, startling unwitting shoppers. An improvisation. Picture him injecting doubt into the audience's mind: none of this might be true. See him slinking off the stage. Deterritorializing himself.

The Stand on that Monday night was, as Jackson describes, an encounter of and in 'milieus', where milieus are comprised of "qualities, substances, powers, and events":[128]

> We travel through milieus, and as we pass through them, we pick up bits and pieces (or components) to assemble territories. In this sense, even the body is a milieu—a passage or a phase. . . . Milieus are made of activities and spaces, and ongoing movement among milieus creates territories.[129]

Milieus are fluid, processual, multiple and can be seen to be composed of "a series of submilieus".[130] Pete, each of us, with our histories and hopes, that basement room, the alcohol, the mic, that particular Monday evening in January, 2016: milieus and submilieus that "[had] no apparent function until these heterogeneities contingently encounter each other and communicate".[131] 'Rhythm', Jackson goes on to say, is the "creative act" that enables "connections with and within (and between and among) milieus, and rhythms that are not too repetitive become *expressive*".[132] Refrains are rhythmic: "Rhythm is in the in-between space—the intermilieu where *difference* is generated".[133] The refrain works in the threshold, at the edge of disorder. It is not the repetition of the same; the refrain is rhythmic, not metric, not the irritating tapping of a pen on a table top, as Jackson suggests, nor the 'earworm', the repetitive fragment of a banal popular song that we cannot shake off. The refrain produces difference.

Pete has performed this set before, even if only in the privacy of his kitchen, speaking into a hairbrush to an audience of plants and cats outside the window. Yet he has never performed this set before. Not here, not this evening. The audience has experienced comedy before, in some form or another. They know what happens. Yet they have never witnessed this before. They have been to the supermarket before. Yet they will not walk their trolley along the fresh produce aisle the same way tomorrow. They have felt sad. They go to a doctor. They believed Pete went to a doctor. They know that claims for 'truth' are suspended here. I believed he went to the doctor. I did not know this would happen.

Surprise is the springing of the familiar into different awareness, a sudden, slant look at what's known: we have been here before and recognize it for the very first time.[134] Surprise is an emergence, an irruption, a "de-phasing", as Erin Manning would put it: "an instance where the complex nodes of incipient relation tune toward what can be singled out as a discrete iteration: toward a remarkable point".[135] The refrain is—I reach towards this, uncertain—the condition of such emergence of surprise: the reaching out of chaos, a momentary claim to territory, an opening to other possibilities. Surprise irrupts in the threshold.

Refrains do not make everything possible. They are not limitless. With their albeit hesitant territorial claim they close other possibilities. Pete's exit, in his sudden departure from the stage, makes some things possible and others not. He introduces doubt. What can we trust? Trust becomes something else. Refrains refrain. They hold back, close down. "Refrains", write Bertelsen and Murphie, "constitute what will always be fragile . . . territories in time. These allow new forms of expression but render others inexpressible".[136] And what is made possible, or not, is not always welcome or easy. Surprise can be uncomfortable.

The refrain is an ontological process of the rhythmic production of difference. My argument is not for the Deleuzoguattarian refrain being synonymous with surprise but for surprise as an 'accompaniment' to the refrain, an affective surge harnessed by it; perhaps even for surprise as being *of* the refrain. The metric dripping of the pipe outside my window does not surprise, but the backflip of Jackson's paper was the rhythmic emergence of difference amongst repetition and it 'caught' the moment by surprise. At Red Raw, that Monday evening, difference emerged amongst the familiarity of a crowd, of bodies compressed, the energetic, pacing demeanour of an upbeat MC, the drudge of yet another series of male comics talking about failed sex, and we found ourselves with Pete lobbing lemons in Aldi.

SURPRISE, THE REFRAIN AND WRITING-AS-INQUIRY

Writing here on what is for now page 42 of this draft text, in single-spaced, Arial size 11 font, this early morning—writing about Pete and his supermarket fruit, typing a way into considering how stand-up might help us think about, understand and undertake writing-as-inquiry—wondering whether the link is going to be there or whether I've taken it as far as it will go—I find the refrain. Or the refrain finds me, seeks me out, finds me again; and, with it, despite my looking for it, surprise. Not surprise as 'method', not surprise as research tool, not surprise as action and intention, but surprise as event. Surprise as excess. A "bloom space".[137] A bloom space that could take us anywhere. A bloom space with options.

> A bloom space can catch you up and then deflate, pop, leave you standing, a fish out of water. Or, same thing, it can catch you in its moves. . . . A bloom space is pulled into being by the tracks of refrains that etch out a way of living in the face of everything. These refrains stretch across everything, linking things, sensing them out—a worlding. Every refrain has its gradients, valences, moods, sensations, tempos, elements, and life spans.[138]

The gradients here, now, at my desk, might be steep, the moods uncertain, the sensations painful. Writing-as-inquiry is a worlding, a creative-relational irruption, that risks rendering us immobile, a fish out of water. Writing's uncertainty, its edge, its between-ness, we both value and avoid.

We tell ourselves we are searching for the new; we say we do not want to find what we already know. We say we want to write into the "not yet known", as Ken Gale and I claim.[139] We tell ourselves this. I tell myself this. But I do and I don't. I want to be in a state of unknowing only some of the time. Sometimes, I may be ready to be surprised; sometimes, I am open to what I have never considered, never understood, never known, but it's not what I always want.

There may be what Cixous terms "happy accidents"[140] but becoming open to the new is arduous. Writing to the rhythm of the refrain in that in-between space, the *intermilieu*—there, at the edges of disorder, in the threshold where difference is generated—Pete and his audience at the The Stand as he disappears from the stage—writing like that, there, is troubling. It might leave you standing. Yet writing there, to the rhythm of the refrain, in the threshold, is where inquiry happens:

> I don't know what to make of thresholds, and I'm not sure whether I like them, but my intuition, my gut, tells me it's where our research needs to be. I want to push thresholds . . . towards a place—a multiplicity of spaces and times—where categories (this and that, here and there) become indistinct, where we position ourselves and our inquiries as always in thresholds, forever liminal, forever refusing "here" or "there," seeking out the pauses, not the notes, in the song; the pauses as notes. In such thresholds our research can be at its most critical, where we take nothing for granted, where everything is at stake. It means conducting inquiries as if we do not know where they will take us. As if there were no more time.[141]

Easy to say, I now think. Easier to assert than to embody. Perhaps most of us, most of the time, tend towards the familiar, the striated, but when we allow refrains to carry us into and through that intermilieu, writing-to-inquire can perhaps become close to how Derrida describes Foucault's work, as carrying a question within it, "a question that keeps [us] in suspense, holding [our] breath—and, thus, keeps [us] alive".[142] Not the kind of formulaic 'research question' funders demand of us and we may demand of our students. Such questions don't hold their breath; they position themselves within neo-liberal discourse as 'useful' and 'relevant', telling us of their potential for generating 'impact'. No, not that; instead the refrains of writing-to-inquire might take us into questions that are "provocative, risky, stunning, astounding. . ., [that take] our breath away with [their] daring".[143] Inquiry that surprises. Inquiry that gives us butterflies. Inquiry that gives us goose bumps. Inquiry that troubles.

With writing-as-inquiry, if we take Laurel Richardson, Elizabeth St Pierre and others seriously, we do not know what will happen when we begin to write. I sometimes do not register how radical this proposal for writing-as-inquiry itself is, given the over-coded, molar norms of academic writing that prevail.[144] Nor how arduous, how intimidating, how—sometimes—terrifying it is. We open the laptop on our desk at home or take out our notebook on a train and, if we are writing to inquire, we *do not know what will happen*. It is the refrain, the gathering of the familiar, the search for rhythm, the "cutting edge of deterritorialisation".[145] We do not know what we will find, what will emerge, what will irrupt, what we will become in touch with. We have to become familiar with that sense of fingers being suspended over keys, uncertain, not knowing what will be next.

In writing to inquire on another early winter morning, just as in the audience at The Stand on that Monday evening, refrains are at work. Refrains bring surprise. No, perhaps it is better to say they create the conditions of possibility for surprise. Refrains and surprise are inseparable. Implicated. Coupled. Refrains carry surprise on their shoulders. It is 7.05am and still dark outside. I am in our back room at my desk. I have been here for thirty minutes, trying to find words. Our son is asleep downstairs. I worry for him; I wonder what will become of him. He—this—is with me as I write. He will find his way in. It's inevitable. Looking up and out of the sash window, I see the glow of a hidden streetlight on the sidewall of a low block of tenements, the kick of a lofted ball away. The throw of a lofted lemon. Beyond that wall, a seven-story tenement block rises. One room on the top floor is lit. Someone is awake; someone has work to get up for; someone has a baby to feed, a child demanding breakfast, an elderly parent needing help. Just this one lit room. Surely there must be other people rising? Don't other people also have to get up to go to work, also have children, also have commitments? The roof of the tenement block is pierced by multiple chimneys that open to an easing sky beginning to reveal its blue, a rare clear day summoned.

These are the milieus and submilieus of this morning's writing-to-inquire: the spread of courtyards, trees and apartments; my desk, its two piles of books, the family photos stuck to the wall above; this room, the window's open shutters, sofa, clutter; the Jonathan-in-process of the morning; the technology of silver laptop and black keys. Our lad, downstairs, hurt, recovering. These are the milieus and submilieus that are looking to connect, "nuclei of eternity lodged between instants".[146] We have been here before, all of us, all of this. We do this every morning. This is our daily appointment with each other. This is our familiar, repeated encounter, where nothing might happen, but where something also might. This is where the tap-tap-tapping of fingers on keys might find rhythm not metre. This, the refrain, is not about 'waiting for inspiration'. This is not glamorous, not the romantic fantasy of the writing appearing, fully wrought and devastating. This is mundane, everyday, every day, plodding, a slog. Deleuze and Guattari write of the refrain:

> One ventures from home on the thread of a tune. Along sonorous, gestural, motor lines that mark the customary path . . . and graft themselves onto or begin to bud 'lines of drift' with different loops, knots, speeds, movements, gestures, and sonorities.[147]

Writing-as-inquiry is a venture from home on the thread of a tune, looking for and open to that which might glide away from the familiar. Like Pete and the audience, when we know he is nearing the end of his set, and he hesitates at the mic before saying, "Of course, none of this might be true".

Surprise is not always welcome, even if it is what we need:

> Writing: a way of leaving no space for death, of pushing back forgetfulness, of never letting oneself be surprised by the abyss. Of never becoming resigned, consoled; never turning over in bed to face the wall and drift asleep again as if nothing had happened; as if nothing could happen.[148]

Writing is a process that can enable us to push back the limits of what we are able contemplate, to test the limits of what we can lose. Cixous is suggesting it is writing that takes us to these experiences so that we might not otherwise be surprised. Writing takes us close to death, to forgetfulness, to the abyss, so we will not be surprised, so we will never become complacent. Who wants to be surprised by an abyss? But we write because we want to live, we are willing to go where it leads, wherever that may be, to take the line of flight that the refrain makes possible. Rolling over in bed to face the wall and allowing ourselves to snooze is enticing but dull.

Perhaps what Cixous is implying here is that writing-to-inquire makes it possible for us to become in touch with that which is unconscious, out of sight.[149] Patricia Clough speaks of something similar when she casts her writings as 'experimental compositions' that seek both to engage and to evoke unconscious processes.[150] In such a psychoanalytic understanding, writing offers the possibility that we will get taken close to that which is most hidden, most out of reach. In the abyss of our unconscious is the violence and destructiveness, the rage and envy, but also the unrequited longing and hope, and (for Deleuze and Guattari, if not for Cixous) the creative possibilities, the productiveness, we are unable—yet—to contemplate. We keep them there, apparently locked away, in our anxiety that, were we to allow them air, they might overwhelm us and perhaps harm ourselves or others. The abyss of which she speaks is the horror of what we keep hidden from ourselves, the spectre of what could engulf. (Now, I hesitate; especially now. The words will not come. This paragraph has taken longer than any other to write thus far. Writing, I am not sure what I will find and I am not sure that I will like it.)

Ah, yes, but then I catch myself. "[I]t's romantic, isn't it?", Sophie Tamas asks about writing. "Edgy. As if anything truly dangerous is ever going to happen in a scholarly journal".[151] Cixous—and now me—may be taking both ourselves and writing too seriously.

The view of the unconscious (and there are many views) I have suggested above the risks portraying affect as being contained within the body, individual, whereas the capture of a moment in writing, even at the break of dawn alone at a desk, is a collaborative act.[152] Even alone I am in relation. Even alone I am of the Deleuzoguattrian event. "Affect", writes Erin Manning,

> is [collective. It] propulses individuation at the between where all projects are most volatile, where group-subjects falter, where the actually living intersect with the already-undead of life's immanent surface. Always more than one, affect creates 'holes of individuality' that animate *a life*.[153]

So the act of writing-to-inquire may perhaps be better understood as being attuned to what might be emerging. Rather than dropping a rope into the nethermost reaches of an unfathomable pit, it is an act of being still on the surface of the ocean, waiting to sense where the waves carry us. Writing-as-inquiry as indeterminacy. "In/determinacy is an always already opening up-to-come", writes Karen Barad. "In/determinacy is the surprise, the interruption, by the stranger (within) re-turning unannounced".[154]

***

In the milieus and intermilieus of the darkened, sweaty comedy club, when the rhythm of the refrain lifts us somewhere different, and the affective rush takes the momentary form of surprise—when that *happens*—we know why we've given up the warmth of our sofa for the evening. Writing, wherever that may be, at whatever time of day, we whistle in the dark, we keep typing. In the milieus and intermilieus of the writing 'field', we might find ourselves—there, then—considering: considering through the keys what we might not have considered in that particular way, and the familiar reveals its strangeness; the refrain carries us. This is where writing-as-inquiry might echo stand-up: not techniques, not methods, but the creation in our inquiries and in ourselves of an attentiveness to the refrain, a capacity to be swept away by the surge of the unexpected and the surprising. Creative-relational inquiry.

MONDAY, 11 JANUARY 2016, RED RAW

The second interval arrives. Three more acts have come and gone since Pete and the first interval. The Wee Man has sent us to the bar to re-fuel. An entwined couple have positioned themselves next to the pillar in front of me and now I can't see the stage.

I am done. Someone else can have my prize spot in this corner by the bar. Not even the excitement of the as-yet-unannounced headline act is enough to keep me. As I pass through the bar, I nod goodbye to Pete. He's talking with a tall young woman with tied-back auburn hair, jeans and black jacket, holding her scarf as if she too is about to leave. I hear her saying, "But a peach would be messier, more fun, wouldn't it?" I leave them and open the door outside. I stand in the porch. Rain falls. It's a ten-minute walk home and whatever I do I'll be sodden by the time I arrive. I wrap my coat around me, pull up my hood, hunch my shoulders, and collect myself for the charge down the hill.

A gutter above is leaking. Drops beat steady onto the lowest step up back to the road. Pah. Pah. Pah. Metre, not rhythm. Time to go.

NOTES

112 Manning, *Always More Than One*, 2013.

113 Hunter, "Reginald D. Hunter Live", 2011.

114 Double, *Getting the Joke*, 2013; Allen, *Attitude*, 2001.

115 Lee, *If You Wanted a Milder Comedian*, 2011, 325.

116 Berlant and Ngai, "Comedy Has Issues", 2017.

117 Massumi, "The Autonomy of Affect", 1995.

118 Dosse, *Intersecting Lives*, 2010.

119 Jackson, "An Ontology of a Backflip", 2016.

120 Jackson, 185.

121 Deleuze and Guattari, *A Thousand Plateaus*, 2004.

122 Jackson, "An Ontology of a Backflip", 2016, 184.

123 Jackson, 184.

124 Jackson, 184.

125 Barad, "Diffracting Diffraction", 2014.

126 Jackson, "An Ontology of a Backflip", 2016, 185.

127 In Boutang, "L'Abécédaire de Gilles Deleuze", 1988.

128 Deleuze, *Essays Critical and Clinical*, 1998, 61.

129 Jackson, "An Ontology of a Backflip", 2016, 186.

130 Jackson, 186, drawing upon Bogue, *Deleuze on Music, Painting and the Arts*, 2003.

131 Jackson, 186.

132 Jackson, 186, emphasis in the original.

133 Jackson, 187.

134 Eliot, *Four Quartets*, 2009.

135 Manning, *Always More Than One*, 2013, 18.

136 Bertelson and Murphie, "An Ethics of Everyday Infinities and Powers", 2010, 139.

137 Stewart, "Worlding Refrains", 2010.

138 Stewart, 342.

139 Wyatt and Gale, "Writing to It", 2018.

140 In Sellars, *The Writing Notebooks of Hélène Cixous*, 2004, ix.

141 Wyatt, "Always in Thresholds", 2014, 16.

142 Derrida, *The Work of Mourning*, 2003, 88.

143 St. Pierre, "Post Qualitative Research", 2011, 623.

144 See Aitchison and Lee, "Research Writing", 2007.

145 Deleuze and Guattari, *A Thousand Plateaus*, 2004, 371.

146 Guattari, *Chaosmosis*, 1995, 17.

147 Deleuze and Guattari, *A Thousand Plateaus*, 2004, 344.

148 Cixous, *Coming to Writing*, 1991, 3.

149 Sellers, *The Writing Notebooks of Hélène Cixous*, 2004.

150 Clough, *The User Unconscious*, 2018.

151 Tamas and Wyatt, "Telling", 2013, 61.

152 And not only human collaboration. See Clough, *The User Unconscious*, 2018, and her argument for an unconscious expanded beyond the 'subject' through digital media and computational technologies into the vibrancy of the other-

than-human. A conceptualizing of the unconscious as relational, dispersed and/or collective (if not in line with Clough's particular take) is one widely embraced within psychodynamic discourse, and also by Deleuze and Guattari. See also note 34 of Interval: Towards Creative-Relational Inquiry (2): The Problem and Promise of the Personal regarding Patricia Clough's troubling of what we mean by 'the body'.

153 Manning, "Always More Than One", 2010, 126. Emphasis in the original.
154 Barad, "Diffracting Diffraction", 2014, 178.

CHAPTER 5

THE REFRAINS OF THERAPY AND THE EVERYDAY

Edinburgh, Spring 2018

The refrain has stayed with me since witnessing Pete at Red Raw and writing the previous chapter some two years ago. Here, I work further with the refrain, searching for it as it arises both in therapy and in the everyday, in the ordinary of living. The writing in this chapter is impressionistic, tentative, incommensurate. Writing it has felt like a dreaming with and of the refrain. The chapter "[moves] in the direction of the incomplete".[155]

Early March 2018. It's over two years since Pete and The Stand. Like all of the UK and much of Europe, Edinburgh has been in the vice grip of an apparently apocalyptic cold spell that, in the UK's case, brought everything to a halt. My university shut down for three days; cafés and shops closed, with signs in their windows stating the obvious. However, one read: "Winter has come. We warned you. Back when we've fought off the white walkers. Love, Jon Snow. PS Wish us luck".[156]

Yesterday, no snow fell and the cold began to ease. The thaw is slow, the dying white blanket stained and ugly; speared icicles melt from the gutters outside my window, dripping at long regular intervals. Pah. Pah. Pah.

Mum is onto her third infection of the past month, though yesterday's news was good: she was well enough to have gin and tonic before Sunday lunch. Tomorrow, I travel south just for the day to visit her. I haven't seen her since November.

For two years I have been searching for refrains. I have been looking, listening, yearning, for them since that Monday night at the The Stand and Pete. I have been seeking refrains in everything, from the mundane of everyday life—work, home, travelling, family, sleeping—to the apparent mundane of therapeutic work: greet, walk, sit, talk.

In February I gave a presentation about the refrain at a conference in India to a room full of therapists. In my presentation I brought the audience into my thinking about how I, perhaps we, might think, live and undertake therapeutic work with the refrain; what the concept of the refrain might offer us, what it might open up. My talk was impressionistic, open-ended, allusive, with slides showing images of comedy clubs and consulting rooms. There was limited text and few bullet points. I thought my talk went well.

The next morning, an eminent professor (I know this because she told me) stopped me at the entrance to the conference building. She was not alone. She had three PhD students in tow, each of whom she introduced and each of whose PhD projects she summarized for me. The students did not speak but each greeted me with a smile. The glass rotating door behind the professor was now blocked by her and her troop. Introductions complete, she turned to me and asked,

So, what was it you wanted to tell us in your presentation yesterday morning? What did you want us to take from it?

The refrain has been enchanting me, I wanted to say. Didn't you find it so? But that sounded unconvincing and insufficient and I doubted she would be satisfied. Instead, I replied:

It was about how we might pay attention, different attention, to the detail of what happens with our clients". I was making gestures of precision with my hands. "I wanted to offer a way into that kind of attentiveness"—thumbs and first fingers of each hand together, for emphasis—"something fresh, through Deleuze and Guattari's concept of the refrain.

"Hmm. I see". She began to turn away, then added, looking back, "That wasn't apparent yesterday".

"I'm glad it was just now, at least", I called.

A car pulled up and the driver came round to open the rear door for her. "Come on, girls. Let's go". Two stepped in beside her, the third got in the front.

I watched them drive away.

SEARCHING FOR EVERYDAY REFRAINS (1)

First, some fragments, glimpses, moments, told in the second person, as if. As if they could be not-me, could be more-than, are always more-than; as if they could be *this*:

Like, how the wind finds its way through a closed window, dragging the kitchen door shut. You know this will happen but, refusing to believe, you leave the door ajar each time, in hope.

How coffee cradles in the cup, how its surface speaks of love, hiding its secrets and its politics, how it enters the body as you look, as you listen, as you smell, as you taste; familiar, quotidian, sharp.

How the bus idles at the lights. It pulses, like a dog breathing after a chase. The bus with its mouth open, panting, till the lights return to green and there are more stops to catch.

The indistinct quiet of early morning. The strands of the palm in front of the window, swaying at its ends in the breeze. You watch and wait. It's like the strands hear a call from a distance and twist, rock, in acknowledgement. A secret message. Call and response.

You cross the square by the National Gallery in late Friday morning winter sunlight on your way up the hill to meet a student. You worry you might be late. For the first time in many days the view east is clear to Arthur's Seat.[157] A busker plays by the wall that overlooks Princes Street gardens. Her hood covers her face, only her mouth visible at the mic. She has a guitar and a small amp and her song is mournful. You want to linger but can't. You reach into your pocket. You have no change.

How she leans against you in the dance, and you turn with each other, shoulders touching, just, around and around. How your hands clasp at the end of the dance, you smile at each other, then each move onto a different dancer, your bodies re-shaped by the print of the other.

***

Deleuze and Guattari's biographer, François Dosse, tells us it was Félix Guattari, of the two of them, who coined—created—the concept of the refrain they take up in *A Thousand Plateaus*:

> [I]n 1979, Guattari wrote a personal text about the refrain, insisting right away that it conjures away the passage of time, the anxiety of death, the risk of chaos, the fear of losing control expressed by *refrains*, these rhythms that produce inhabited, territorialized time.[158]

It was Guattari, the pianist, to whom the refrain came. I imagine their taking it up together in the epistolary way of their early collaborations: Guattari, the psychoanalyst, writing at La Borde, the radical psychiatric clinic near the Loire in which he was immersed for most of his working life,[159] sending his writing to Deleuze in Paris to work and re-work; and how they might have argued over it in their Tuesday afternoon meetings at Deleuze's house, on Guattari's weekly visits to Paris for teaching commitments and to attend Lacan's seminars.

Guattari would write about the refrain in his final work before he died in 1992:

> 'I haven't driven for years'; or, 'I feel like learning word processing'. A remark
> of this kind may remain unnoticed in a traditional conception of analysis.
> However, this kind of singularity can become a key, activating a complex
> refrain, which will not only modify the immediate behaviour of the patient,
> but open up new fields of virtuality for him: . . . Respond to the event as the
> potential bearer of new constellations of Universes of reference.[160]

Respond, he seems to suggest, with Alecia Jackson, to the rhythm. Feel the connections with, within, between, among milieus. Listen, sense, if you can, for those in-between spaces where difference is produced.

The everyday—like a young woman performing a backflip at a sporting event,[161] like a comedy performer on a Monday evening—might offer such refrains.

What might be present when the door always closes in the draught, or a bus pauses at the lights? What might be happening in the sway of leaves in the wind, in hearing the busker's song, in a dance encounter, or in coffee and its unspoken? Can I pay attention? Where is the rhythm? Is there rhythm? Can I *feel* it? Can I sense the "nuclei of eternity lodged between instants"?[162] I think I can, sometimes: walking past the busker, there was a moment of transport. It wasn't just the song, wasn't just the phrasing of her voice. It was the sense of being on the cusp, caught, in the possible. In what could be, as I kept walking, as I took one more step away, as I felt for change and found none.

SEARCHING FOR THERAPY REFRAINS (1)

"A remark of this kind . . . can become a key, activating a complex refrain", Guattari writes. 'Remarks' may not be spoken, may not be verbal. They may be present, but unsaid. Or offered, enacted.[163] A gesture here, a movement there. Not "I haven't driven for years" but how this evening Karl reaches for his bottle of water on the side, the clear blue plastic bottle he places there each week before he sits. He reaches out his hand, some ten minutes into the session as silence settles. He does this. The movement is wallpaper, or 'ground' perhaps, but this time he hesitates, a halt as he touches the blue with his finger, and the move jolts into awareness, into 'figure'.[164] I wasn't looking, I wasn't watching, but the break caught me.

'Remarks' of this kind may sometimes be noticed but they may remain overlooked, even when we're alert. And even when they do make themselves known, any "new constellations" may be hard to imagine. That momentary stillness, that singularity, of finger on bottle: it may be nothing. But I hope, as does Guattari: I see it as if it *could be* something. I try to allow myself to be open, though rhythm is so difficult to sense and refrains so elusive.

Or like:[165]
This is not how Karl imagined it would be, not what he'd hoped. The way the days keep rolling, one into the other.

He lies in bed when it's time to get up.

He makes the same breakfast each morning. Cereal, fruit, tea. He knows the precise amounts of each. He knows which order he will place them in his bowl.

He knows how each of the others takes their tea: no milk, no sugar; milk, one sugar; milk, no sugar. Of course. Who wouldn't know after all this time? Is that what love is now? Is that loyalty? Habit?

It's all he can do to talk to her. It takes too much from him. The pain rises as he feels his voice. Staying quiet keeps him numb, but it feels a sort of peace.

Or like:
I'm tired.

Ally is a big woman. Her size is what has brought her to therapy. She reports to me how she is unable to find the energy to cook for herself so she eats takeaways most nights.

I'm tired.

She tries to exercise but getting on the exercise bike at home in her flat is dull and joining a gym—or joining anything—is a horrifying prospect.

I'm tired.

We walk the corridor, she enters the room behind me, takes off her coat, removes the cushion from the chair, sits, sighs, and opens:

I'm tired.

How, before it's time to begin, the room, room 4, has to be re-arranged. The window opened, circulation allowed. Chairs like this: not too close, not too far; angled, at a slight tilt. Seductive, almost. Lamps switched on. One, two, three, in turn: by the door, on the table between the chairs, in the far corner. Overhead light off: too bright, too obvious. Instead, the soft, warm lamplight. Seductive, almost. With five minutes to go, I kneel on the hard-carpeted floor, chest to knees, forehead resting on the ground, hands outstretched. Child pose. Breathing slow and deep, trying to let go of all else but this. Gradual rise to my feet. Now.

(Note: I use the first and third person, not second person, in these therapy moments. As I write I find both the 'other', the particular other, and the singular, if provisional, 'I', have to be present. It's a matter of politics.[166])

How, in the counsellors' office each Tuesday evening, as we make tea and notes, and as we watch the clock on the wall nudge towards the hour, we observe who is and who is not in the Stripy-Socked Counsellors' Club. We imagine it as an indicator (or otherwise) of the depth of our insight and skill as practitioners, and suggest those who are not in the SSCC should take this serious matter to clinical supervision. It's a running joke amongst us, made in those minutes before our clients arrive, when we are none of us quite sure of who we are or what we will become.

How my first therapist lived a in a village a thirty minutes' drive away. On Friday evenings for three years, when the children were small, I would say goodbye as they ate tea and watched TV and I would drive to her home at 7.00pm. Fields sloped uphill to the right as I turned into her road. I would park up outside her semi-detached house on a 1970s estate at the edge of the village.

Inside the wooden and glass front door, I'd follow her along the short corridor, treading the worn, wine-red, patterned carpet to a room on the left, enter and sit on the far chair. Sometimes—for weeks at one point—I would lie on the couch that ran along one wall. One time I lay the whole hour in silence, clutching a soft toy. She didn't interrupt. She stayed. I opened my eyes and she was there, unmoving and watchful.

But most times I would sit in the chair and I would talk, trying to make progress.

On the way to her house I would listen to the news. On the journey home the same weekly Michael Parkinson radio programme would be on and over the sound of the engine I would listen to his gentle conversations with sports stars and not to the sounds of my body and whichever of my own conversations I was conducting.

***

In this searching—as Karl makes his routine morning tea, as another client speaks of her fatigue, as I adjust the lighting, as I call out the plain sock wearers, as I remember my Friday evening journey to see my therapist—I scroll back a few pages, reminding myself how refrains are always about territory, always about the processes of entering and exiting territory. Which, in turn, takes me to the red ship.

Bertelson and Murphie bring their readers into a moment in 2001 when a red Norwegian freighter carrying 438 rescued, mostly Afghani, refugees entered Australian territorial waters.[167] The authors show us this moment and what ensued, inviting us to consider the image of this vast red hulk as a refrain that found its way into the affective everyday of Australian political and cultural life. They describe how the entry of the *Tampa* into Australian waters, its takeover by troops, and the transporting of the asylum seekers aboard to the island of Nauru, marked a shift in the Australian government's handling of such refugees. It is a story of who was (and continues to be) allowed in and who was (and continues to be) kept out. From that point, from the red ship onward, refugees entering by sea would be taken to Nauru or alternatively to Papua New Guinea, both of which were in turn handed generous Australian government re-imbursements.

At the moment of crossing into Australian territory, the red ship became the refrain, the "mark",[168] of the new territory that emerged in this unfolding Deleuzoguattraian 'event' (a collective something-that-happens), an event that in turn opened onto the possibility of further events and new territories that were both physical (e.g. detention centres) and existential (discourses, laws, modes of living, etc.): "In sum, a new field of expression [arose], a refrain that [potentialized] other refrains".[169] The red ship—vast, persistent, material—was the refrain carried in the press and on TV, a refrain suggestive of conflict, anxiety and ambiguity (did the *Tampa* convey threat or humanitarian need or both?).

79

Bertelson and Murphie invoke psychoanalyst Daniel Stern's notion of the red ship's "temporal contour"[170]—its specificity, its particular moment—intersecting with the temporal contour of 9/11, which happened a matter of weeks later. At this intersection, because of this intersection, long-lasting, reactionary, authoritarian state responses and polarizing, aggressive discourses followed, "the red ship refrain now bleeding into what was become a culture entrained to be wary of anything that hinted at 'softness'".[171] The red ship, the refrain of the red ship, opened onto and into other territories and made other refrains possible that, in this case, gave rise to oppressive courses of action, not only in relation to asylum seekers but arguably stretching to the demeaning and scapegoating of other marginalized, excluded others within and beyond Australia at the time.

So here is one reason for dwelling with Bertelson and Murphie's text and the red ship: not all refrains are desirable (depending upon your position), not all refrains open onto new territory that is ethical and progressive (depending upon your position). Any searching for refrains needs to be able to discriminate and be alert: "the economy of collective desire goes both ways, in the direction of transformation and liberation, and in the directions of paranoic wills to power".[172]

Which leads to a second point: how any refrain-yearning on my part needs to understand how none of what transpired in this episode was inevitable. There were other outcomes possible when the *Tampa* appeared on the Australian horizon. The refrain is unpredictable, transitional, and imbued with power:

> The form of a refrain is not, therefore, a stable distribution of 'formed' affects. It is an erratic and evolving distribution of both coming into being and the power to affect or be affected. This is its power. The refrain is a particularly useful way of negotiating the relations between everyday infinities of virtual potentials and the real (that is, not just theorized) operations of power. Refrains enable modes of living in time, not in 'states'.[173]

I arrange the lighting in room 4 each week. There's routine to it, maybe even a rhythm to it (how it acts between worlds, mine and my soon-to-arrive client): the pressing of switches, my steps from one to the next, my standing and looking around to check. It's a series of actions that goes along with adjusting the cushions, emptying the bin, and opening the window. It's about care. It's about comfort. It's about preparation. But it's not only these. "Seductive, almost", I write earlier. The acts are neither innocent nor neutral. They may be undertaken with the best of conscious intentions but they operate between "everyday infinities and real . . . operations of power".

In my continuing search for refrains I have to remember how the refrain is inherently pragmatic rather than ethical, the feature of ethical refrains being their preservation of a sense of uncertainty, "an opening to affective infinities and powers, while making the affective more livable"[174] When I hold the door open for my client, and they walk into a soft-lit room, something might happen, beyond intention, beyond doing, beyond knowing.

Beyond knowing, because the red ship refrain, carried on its specific temporal contour, evoked live, fluid affective responses that were sensed but not named. Such unconscious affective responses Stern terms 'vitality affects'—"shifts in internal states"[175]—in contrast to the more defined 'categorical affects' (known emotions, those we might name, like anger). The red ship refrain turns like the ship itself, and comes into relation with other temporal contours—9/11—and their associated vitality affects, in unstable relation between different intensities, different speeds, a *simple* refrain complexifying[176]—the red ship, pictures of the Australian prime minister, the national flag, etc.—and the affective wave of these complex refrains prompting multiple, often contradictory, social and political responses and actions. Karl reaches for his water bottle, the clear blue plastic bottle he places there each week before he sits. He reaches out his hand, some ten minutes into the session as silence settles, and hesitates. The hesitation catches me. It's just a sense, that's all. But it's a sense that may bring us into relation, for good or ill or both, with as-yet unknown territories.

ASIDE: RETURN TO RED RAW, SEARCHING FOR STAND-UP REFRAINS

Ryan Cullen, the first performer, has a soft Irish accent that lulls you. His friend stood next to me as we waited for the start of the show, poised to take photos of him when he strode on stage. However, the spot she'd chosen was empty for a reason, given that the pillar obscured her view of the stage, but she stayed to warn me that Cullen is dark. His gigs are well received in Ireland, she said, but somehow don't seem to go down well in

Scotland. She seemed puzzled and a little hurt as she made this observation, looking up at me as if I might have an explanation. A few minutes later she disappeared.

Cullen's opening line is: "It's a good thing I watched Bambi as a kid. It made watching my mother get shot much easier". We laugh but the laugh does not last long and has no great pleasure within it. I can see what she meant about dark, and about how he might not go down well. Not all surprise is good; not all surprise does the work that I am interested in. Later in the set he tells us: "How embarrassing it is to watch sex scenes on TV with your parents. I think, why did they have to film themselves?" When he finishes, I take out my notebook so as to not lose this line, unsure what to make of it. The trouble I have is not with the lines themselves, which are clever and well-wrought. It's just that I find myself not caring.

Whereas, with Tom Joyce, I care from the moment he walks on stage. I care because, for at least the first five of his fifteen minutes I worry about him. He is awkward and shy, mumbling into the mic, removing his sweater over his head, a move that knocks his glasses askew and lifts his shirt to reveal a bulging hairy belly. He shuffles, pulling up his trousers, not bothering to re-arrange his hair. He seems like he has stumbled on stage by mistake, on his way home to his bedsit after a day spotting trains. When, after what feels too long for comfort, he begins in earnest, he calls on the audience to help him make a better entrance. "So, I'll start again—I'll be at the back of the stage—then you call out 'He looks too relaxed', then one of you says, 'I'm glad he's not my bus driver', to which another one of you will respond, "People like you make me so angry. I'm going to the bar to get a hot dog". Then the bar staff will go, 'We don't do hot dogs' and then you'll shout, 'Well, I'm just going to leave' and storm out. Got it?" He walks us through this scenario once more, pausing to recruit the first volunteer we need, then we do it. We all shout "He looks too relaxed", and a guy in the third row calls out that he's glad Joyce is not his bus driver, then there's hesitancy when no one seems willing to do the angry, hot dog, storming out section, but Joyce cajoles us and the first guy's friend stands, looking reluctant but not unhappy, and he's off, doing a convincing impression of someone who is so outraged he ends up leaving. Joyce has us now. I am no longer worried for him.

SEARCHING FOR EVERYDAY REFRAINS (2)

Again: can I sense the "nuclei of eternity lodged between instants"?[177] Stay longer, I tell myself. See how 'instants' might—or might not—be found in the drab extraordinary of the everyday.

Two institutional glimpses. Longer glimpses, this time.

One:

It's not that the days are the same, exactly; and it's not that they're dull. Different problems arise and each one needs addressing. They each ask for a response for which you have to find the imagination and energy. You have to work at understanding the uniqueness of this particular situation. You have to consult, diagnose, perhaps reframe, perhaps take action. You know each time it will need you to marshal your attention, and courage, and, well, do the best you can.

It's not monotony that draws the life from you. It's persistence. Like the burglar alarm that sounds along the street as you write, just within earshot. You can block out its call for a time as you focus on something else, on this, on writing, but it's there when you lift your head. Always there.

Two:

The meeting is in a top floor room with a view to Salisbury Crags, though the windows are clouded, the vista obscured though you know it's there. Escape is not possible.

On the meeting's agenda are resources, workload, another set of imposed academic institutional requirements, and yet another revision of bureaucratic processes.

It's not a room we're accustomed to, not the one where we expected to be. We squeeze around a ragged rectangle of tables. Some of us speak, many don't.

We rehearse the same positions, articulate the same complaints. The fault lines are ones we know well and are there for us to notice, and we no doubt do, but we leave them aside and move on. Now is not the time.

Today we have biscuits. *Today we have naming of parts.*[178] A gesture from the colleague whose request for us to change rooms, making way for him, we agreed to, hence why we're here. The biscuits circulate but not many are taken.

At the end of the meeting, ninety minutes later, when we scatter with relief, no one knows where or to whom the biscuits belong, so we leave them on the table to gaze at the crags.

In the lift three of us stand in silence. When we reach the ground floor and leave the building we go our separate ways, but the meeting is not over, not for me at least. It's present in the weight of my step.

We should find a different word to 'meeting'. Meeting is not what happens.

***

Such longer glimpses don't speak to me of refrains. I read and re-read, remembering, searching for what I might be missing. I become in touch with those episodes' affects again, still, months later. The first—"It's not that the days are the same, exactly"—feels present again today, the 'you' (me) of the text undone by the relentless.

I wonder what Guattari might have sensed that I am unable to make contact with. I wonder what I, they, any of those in those vignettes, might do differently, what might unlock the apparent stasis, what might need to happen to give rise to 'expression'.

"The refrain", writes Dosse, "also signals the departure for deterritorialization, a change of scenery, a trip, a back and forth between departure and the return, which sets the tone of an in-between of two territories".[179] The meeting's literal "change of scenery" might have offered a different tone but didn't seem to. "[The refrain's] very circularity", continues Dosse, "evokes the fact that there is neither beginning nor end—only infinite variations". Sameness, familiarity, is an illusion. Perhaps when we hear only metre we're missing the rhythm. The signal, the opportunity, for 'departure' is obscured, like the view of the crags. We hold back from noticing because of what it might cost. We might move back and forth, for a moment. We might experiment with the in-between, but we hesitate. The refrain, and its potential "new fields of virtuality" and "new constellations of Universes of reference", may be too daunting. The new and its uncertainty, and its potential scale, can be a fearful prospect.

***

Further everyday instants.

First, a dream:

I dreamt of my father again last night. It's happening often. He was standing, looking across my vision, from right to left, with his stick against his hip, leaning against a wall. He didn't see me. He didn't speak. He just appeared, in a dream about. . . . I don't know what. In those other recent dreams he has been the same: he has been younger, standing tall: my father, standing, as if the dream is calling me to remember how he was, that he once did stand, that his legs used to hold his weight. My father standing, and standing *still*. His stillness. No shaking of his right wrist and arm, no twisting of his face, which towards the end would remind me of a child chewing with disgust; none of the grimaces and contortions of a Parkinsonian body, none of the pain. Just Dad, standing, still and at ease. In my dreams he never talks. I never hear his voice.

Second instant, a phone conversation:

Mum tells me over the phone, "People ask me if I'm happy. I say, 'happy' isn't the word. The word is 'content'. I am content".

I struggle to get to speak with her. She is either not in the public areas when I call or unable to reach the handset in her room. It's been since her fall in January 2017. She fell twice, the second time following her return from hospital after treatment for the damage from the first. The second time she lay on the floor in her room till her friend came to take the dog out. She does not know how long she waited. She fell because she had still not recovered, but the hospital needed the bed.

Now she has only limited movement in her right arm and is unable to support herself when she walks, so she stays seated until the exercises the physiotherapist prescribes re-connect and strengthen the arm and shoulder. None of us is optimistic this will happen, but we remind her to keep at it.

She has learned to eat with her left hand. She no longer uses her phone and we do not text. I call her using the institution's phone. Beverley or Carol answers. They sound cheerful and they recognize me now. Most times I have to call back.

Each time we do manage to speak, she tells me this, as she has done the past five years, even when she was still in her own home. Happy is not the word. I am content.

Final instant, a walk. Just a walk.[180] Montjaux to Castelnau-Pegayrols, Aveyron, France. July 2017:

The forest path follows a lateral line around a series of steep hills. A single narrow, steep, looping road bisects the route, and I follow it for a few minutes before the path re-appears to the left. It's a sharp turn and I double back on myself as it takes a gradual slope downhill. The sun is high, but the heat is not intense and the wide path is shaded. The track curls to the right and up. For a time as I climb the route is open, without tree cover, curving up and around the hillside. I pause, take water, and turn to feel the sun on my face. I feel a gentle wind and hear the sound of a bell from a field below as cows graze. Flies, urgent, land on skin. Butterflies, some red, some white, whose names I know but can't retrieve, dip, climb, dip again and alight, but only for a moment before making their way.

When the path re-enters the forest, the darkness is sudden, interrupted by shards of light ahead. There is movement and sound everywhere as I walk. A cicada begins to play, to the left above me. I have to stop. I listen. It is all I can do to stand. The cicada's sound pulses, it sings, it calls—none of these words, human analogies, works. It calls me to stand still, that's all I know. It continues, tch-tch-tch-tch, tch-tch-tch, tch-tch-tch, crescendo, diminuendo, crescendo, diminuendo. I take out my phone and record, in a vain, reductive desire to capture, to take it with me. I record a minute. It feels like theft. I fear if I move again it will stop. I move. It continues. Not more than twenty paces further on, I pick up the sound of another, the other side, in the trees down to the right: a different tone, a different rhythm, its pauses longer than the first. Again, I stop and record. Further along, there's a third, different again—faster, more urgent—then a fourth, fifth, sixth and I stand to listen to the cluster of their calls. Astounded.

When I Think of You (Walking from Montjaux to Castelnau-Pegayrols and back)

when I think of you

I feel

the way the warm wind brushes
a curving path one late deep-summer afternoon

how the path's edged stones and grass-full earth
caress the steep hillside

when I think of you

I hear

how the geese ease overhead,
call-gliding, slipping the sky

how the cicadas summon,
their insistent rhythms numberless, unique

when I think of you

I see

how a shoal of butterflies surfs the air-swells
colour-skipping in their playful, restless desire

a stand-still moment, sun on skin,
listening, watching, breathing, the joyous overwhelm

yes, when I think of you

I sense

that turning path
that once-in-a-life-abundant afternoon

SEARCHING FOR THERAPY REFRAINS (2): KARL

Karl seems on edge today. He seems unable to settle. He looks out of
the window, then down to the right armrest and sweeps away a speck of
dust with his fingers. He sighs. I'm looking at him, wondering what it
might be. Where he might be. I haven't seen him like this before. Restless.
Uneasy. The usual sheen of confidence is not there. He seems small. Vulnerable. When we walked up the corridor just now he walked slower than

usual. I am used to him being right behind me, but today he dropped back a few paces. I hardly noticed at the time but I think about it now as I wait for him to speak. I toy with asking him what's going on, but decide against it. I wait. We wait.

I can hear the therapeutic pair next door, Paulo and his client. Not the words themselves but the exchange of intonation and pitch, one then the other, a regular, rhythmic to and fro. An unusual balance, him then her then him then her. Over these many months with Karl I don't remember hearing Paulo or his client at all. Perhaps they're talking dates and times, undertaking a routine transaction (he's away, she's away, when will they next meet). That would explain the even exchange but not that I can hear them. Maybe it's something else. Something mutual and surprising. In there and in here.

"I don't know where to start today", Karl says. A look up at the window. "Well, yes I do, but I don't want to". A look down to the armrest. Another speck flicked off. "It's a bit awkward. I feel awkward. Talking about it. With you".

"You could begin perhaps with telling me about how it's awkward. What might happen. What you worry about in telling me".

"No. No". The second 'no' more decisive than the first. He takes a breath, then: "You're such a therapist".

Not looking at me. It's not a neutral observation: he's not saying 'it's warm this evening' or 'the traffic was bad' or 'our cat is sick'. There's a breath, more a sigh, followed by 'you're such a therapist', a statement uttered with impatience though not without kindness. You're such a therapist but I don't blame you for that. It's what you do. You can't help it.

"I don't want to do that", he continues. "I don't want to tell you about what it's like not telling you and the possibilities of what could befall me if I did. I want just to tell you. To tell myself. To admit it to myself".

"Sure".

Silence. Here and next door. Our window is ajar and there is the rhythm of an early evening in late Spring: the call of a child to her mother a street away, a car pulling out, a dog barking.

He sighs again and then speaks. "It's about sex".

I wasn't expecting this. It wasn't that I thought he would never bring this aspect of his life to therapy and it wasn't as if sex hadn't already (and always) been implicitly present, hidden between the stories of home, the distance between him and Shell, and the separate beds. And he'd been to see Katherine Ryan, after all.[181] No, it was the abruptness I hadn't been expecting. How deliberate this was. It's not like we slipped into this conversation. He'd come knowing it's what he needed to discuss.

"I miss it. I miss sex".

"Yes".

"No. That's not true. I miss missing it. I miss wanting it".

He folds his arms. "I can't remember the last time we had sex, Shell and me. Years. Well, two maybe. And now she's in a different room, and we don't do much of anything together. Let alone touch. The nearest we get is posing for family photos at birthdays or at nephews' and nieces' weddings, when I'll put my arm around her or we'll touch shoulders. But I miss *wanting* it more than anything. I miss the contact. I long for that. The touching. The longing for touch is still there sometimes. But not the. . . . Not the urgency. Not those moments when it's *there*, she's there, you're there, and you feel you must; you both feel you must, like it's the most important thing in the world, nothing else matters, nothing else will do. Like it's all that's left".

"Like it's all that's left?"

"Did I just say that? Oh god. That's embarrassing. How sincere. But there it is. That's what I mean though and it's what I miss. How you forget yourself, and this—you and her—is all there is. As if sex will save me, save us. Save the world".

He stops, looks up, and repeats: "Shell and me having sex will save the world".

A sudden shadow blocks the light from outside. I startle. A cat, a tabby, has appeared at the open window, peering its head into the gap and stepping one paw into the room, looking as if it might join us. I stand up, it turns and springs to the ground, out of sight. I take the couple of steps and push the window closed. Karl does not say anything. I turn back to my chair and he appears not to have noticed. He's looking down; he's motionless. I sit.

"You shouldn't have", he says.

"Shouldn't have what?"

"Scared the cat".

"Oh".

"He was okay being there. He could have come in".

"Maybe".

"He heard the sex talk, that was all. He could have joined in. You should have given him a break. Who's there to listen to him, Mister Therapist, exerting your Therapist powers to decide he shouldn't be here?"

"He gave me a shock and I reacted. I was annoyed with him for interrupting you".

"I wouldn't have minded. I'm pleased he turned up. He might have been able to help out".

"Maybe".

"Anyhow. I bet he doesn't have this happen".

"What does he not have happen?"

He doesn't reply. There's another flick of his fingers on the armrest.

"Well, to be blunt . . ."

Smiles, as if to himself.

"That's not a helpful turn of phrase in the circumstances. 'To be blunt'. Oh dear".

I glimpse the cat leap onto the wall just beyond the window. It turns and sits, looking towards us.

"To be blunt. I don't get hard". Then laughs. "I don't know why that's funny, but it is. I won't try to explain".

"No need. I get it". I'm not laughing.

"Well", he says, "it made it easier to get the words out, in any case".

"You got there, yes".

"It's not that I can't, you know, get hard. I don't think. It's not that. It's just I don't. I look for it, though. I look for the wanting, the desire".

"Of course, yes".

He looks at me. "I'm wondering what you're thinking".

"What I'm thinking or what I'm feeling? What are the possibilities you're considering?"

"I'm wondering if you think I'm sad".

"I imagine you may well be *feeling* sad about this, but that's not what you mean, I assume. No, I don't think you're sad".

"That's good, though I'm not sure I believe you. You said that too easily".

"I don't think you're sad. I think you're searching for your vitality. You've lost touch with it".

"That's one way of putting it, true. I don't feel vital. At all. Not in any sense".

The tabby has returned to sit outside the now-closed window. It's a brave cat, this one, I say to myself. Determined.

"Open the window", Karl says. "No", without waiting for me to respond, "actually, I'll do it". When he moves his gestures are heavy, like he has a weight in his hand as he twists the handle and pushes it open a few inches.

"There", he announces as he sits back down. "Now don't be scared this time", he instructs.

The cat remains where it is, seated, ignoring us, it would seem, refusing the invitation for now. It wasn't startled by Karl. I am, though. What just happened? A minor moment, perhaps but, until now, for all this time, it has been me who's attended to the window (or the lighting, or the temperature—the room's 'climate'). I would consult Karl, or other clients, and notice their comfort or otherwise, or they might say something—"it's cold in here, tonight"—but it would be me that attends to it. Not just now, not on this occasion. It's not about comfort, either, it's about who, or what, joins us.

"So, where was I?", he asks.

"Not feeling vital".

"Oh yes. Wanting to want". That flick gesture on the armrest. "I even— get this—I'm not sure if I can say it—" The cat rises onto its paws and pads towards the gap Karl has provided. "—I even cross the road if I see someone attractive on the other side".

Karl stops to look at me like before, trying to read what I make of this, to sense how I am responding, like he knows how he imagines it sounds. The cat is hesitating by the gap.

"Why did the middle-aged git cross the road?" He waits for me to answer.

"I don't know. Why did the middle-aged git cross the road?"

"Because he saw breasts on the other side".

We don't laugh, either of us.

"It's nothing creepy—", he insists.

"Sure", I say, feeling equivocal. "So, tell me more". I'm responding is if this is only him, not me.

"It's just about proximity—"

"Proximity?" As if, of course, I couldn't possibly want such a thing. As if I would never behave in this way. As if I have no understanding for myself of how this might happen.

"It's just so when we pass I can feel closer to her. To something. To contact".

"To maybe?"

"To what if. Could be. Something else. Something different. Away. Not this. Wanting. Wanted".

"Warmth . . ."

"God, no, stop being so obvious. I mean yes of course but it's not just about the body. Bodies. My body".

"It's always about bodies. How can it not be?"

"Well, okay, maybe. But, anyhow, I don't know if I should feel ashamed. Should I? I feel like it should be shameful, for me or anyone. I don't feel ashamed, but I feel I should do. I mean, how would someone feel if they knew?"

"Knew what?"

"That someone they don't know has crossed the road to be near them, and they'd never know".

Neither of us has noticed the cat leave, but we do now. It's slipped away as we found ourselves walking the city's crowded early summer pavements, poised at the point where Karl sees a space in the traffic and begins to cross, a straight man who's noticed an attractive woman walking towards him on the other side, the longing, the loss and the politics of the moment present in the steps he begins to take.

"As if desire—and desiring desire—is shameful?", I ask. Or even misogynistic, or suggestive of harassment; and this, now, his telling me, a demeaning act of admitting to a secret perversion.

He stops at this. And in the seconds of the pause, of holding, both of us, there is this rapid conversation with myself: I wonder what I mean and if I believe what I've said moments ago, that it's all about bodies; and what is a body anyway? And how of course I recognize exactly what he's describing—yearning, is that it?—yet there seems no way to say so that will offer anything but a collusive invitation to be sad old men together acknowledging and enjoying our secret lusts and how can that be helpful; and before I go anywhere with that he begins again.

"I hope that allowing myself to be near attraction I might find it again"—and in hearing that sentence I realize I've missed the point completely, that he and I are not the same and I need to take my own motivations and losses and regrets somewhere else than here—"and there must be something still there if I even notice. It's not as if when I see people they all flatten into a backdrop of vanilla. Some people seem to have colour. Sometimes it might be men, sometimes women. I don't want to want men but I can notice their vitality. I can be drawn by their beauty—a voice, a style, an energy. I don't want them for myself. Not mostly. Don't seek out proximity in the same way. Or don't seek out the desire for that closeness. Maybe I should try it, see if I can find it there".

"Is that what you want?"

"Nah. Maybe. Not sure I'm that interested to be honest."

I feel a lurch inside, a sudden springing to awareness: he's right. I regret chasing the cat away before. What might our cat have done for the work? What might have happened? Why did I leap to my feet so quickly? Why not let the cat in? Or, at least, why not pause and allow a few moments for us to notice and think together? How come I rushed to shut it out? What was I afraid of? Because I was. There was a stab of fear when it turned its head, ears and whiskers pricked, into the gap, curious. That's what Karl had seen, that's what he was inviting in when he got to his feet when the cat gave us a second chance.

I notice a sudden distance. Karl has become flat to me. A cardboard cut-out placed in a chair. I am distracted by thoughts of how the match (Spurs vs West Brom), in which I have only limited investment, will proceed; by the writing I need to do for the Illinois conference in May; by our Joe, many miles away; by the emails I haven't read and need to respond to. Anything. Anything but here. I have left the room. There's nothing here that holds me. I look at Karl, searching for where we can go.

It's coming up to time. Karl calls me back.

"I'm pleased I talked about this with you today. I never thought I would. I thought I'd never have the courage".

"How has it left you?"

I think, 'that was another therapist cliché', but Karl doesn't call me out for it. He's thoughtful, then responds.

"I'm okay. I'm sad, you're right. That's what it is mostly. I'm just sad, sad, sad".

"Of course. Yes".

"You know what? I'm sad too about the cat not coming in. That's why I wanted it to be here with us. I had this idea he would come and join us.

That he'd want to be with us. Part of this. Part of us. I wanted him to want to be here".

***

"[Therapy's] meaning", says Guattari, "resides in its *processual direction*, in its processual openness, in the refrain, understood . . . in the existential sense of an auto-affirmation".[182] I could interpret Karl's declaration of his loss of libido. I could categorize it as such. I could look for connections between the intruding cat and the loss of his desire. I could look for connections between his loss of desire and the dynamic between the two of us, in the room, the 'transference', how I sense we move in and out of 'contact', how I am perhaps a 'flat' presence to him, as well as he to me, distant 'others' to each other, others we can walk away from.

These thoughts may well take me somewhere. I think these, I wonder these. However, I am closer to how Guattari calls me to see Karl-and-me-and-the-cat-talking-about-desire-and-ethics as the refrain's working within and towards our processual openness. The cat as a refrain, on its particular 'temporal contour', intersecting with that of Karl's hand flicking the arm of his chair—*there*—and others (the counsellor and client next door, their talk-sounds emerging into Karl-and-me-sitting-waiting; bodies that open and close the window) so that *something could happen*. Something creative-relational, opening onto territories that had not been explored, even if only for a moment before we—I—took fright.

Refrains turn and return, create and re-create, emerge and re-emerge, aslant, bearing the potential for new constellations of difference. The way coffee feels, how a door shuts in the wind, a man reaching for his water bottle, how a cat sits by a window.

NOTES

155 Biehl and Lock, "Deleuze and the Anthropology of Becoming", 2010, 319.

156 A reference to the long-running HBO series, *Game of Thrones*.

157 Arthur's Seat is the main peak of a group of hills to the east of Edinburgh city centre.

158 Dosse, *Intersecting Lives*, 2010, 253.

159 Dosse; Boldt and Valente, "L'école Gulliver and La Borde", 2016.

160 Guattari, *Chaosmosis*, 1995, 17–18.

161 Jackson, "An Ontology of a Backflip", 2016.

162 Guattari, *Chaosmosis*, 1995, 17.

163 MacLure, "The Refrain of the A-Grammatical Child", 2016.

164 Goldstein, *The Organism*, 1939.

165 As in the first Interval, I am using 'like', with Manning and Massumi, to convey both particularity and affective excess, suggesting how what follows is not identical but hinting at what is there and/but beyond.

166 See the second Interval, which discusses the politics of the personal pronoun.

167 Bertelson and Murphie, "An Ethics of Everyday Infinities and Powers", 2010.

168 Bertelson and Murphie, 142.

169 Bertelson and Murphie, 142.

170 Bertelson and Murphie; Stern, *The Present Moment*, 2004.

171 Bertelson and Murphie, 143.

172 Guattari, *Soft Subversions*, 2009, 71.

173 Bertelson and Murphie, "An Ethics of Everyday Infinities and Powers", 2010, 145.

174 Bertelson and Murphie, 156.

175 Stern, *The Present Moment*, 2004, 64.

176 Guattari, *Chaosophy*, 2009.

177 Guattari, *Chaosmosis*, 1995, 17.

178 Reed, "Naming of Parts", in *A Map of Verona*, 1946.

179 Dosse, *Intersecting Lives*, 2010, 253.

180 This 'just' is, of course, ironic, as what follows hopefully conveys concerning the power of walking. See Springgay and Truman, *Walking Methodologies*, 2018.

181 See Chapter 3.

182 Ettinger, "From Transference to Aesthetic Paradigm", 2002, 244

Chapter 6

THREE SHITS

A Connection of Some Kind[183]

February–March 2015, Edinburgh

This chapter works and plays with 'ordinary affect', as it flows amongst, through and between three different milieus: my university workplace, a therapeutic encounter with Karl, and a comedy club.

> Ordinary affect is a surging, a rubbing, a connection of some kind that has an impact. It's transpersonal or prepersonal—not about one person's feelings becoming another's but about bodies literally affecting one another and generating intensities: human bodies, discursive bodies, bodies of thought, bodies of water.[184]

Shit One

This morning. My office at the university. Early. Winter. It's dark, but I get the sense of light somewhere beyond, in hiding.

A silent room on a silent corridor. Except I hear the low, slow, relentless hum of the systems that keep this building breathing. Barely: it is a building on life support. It is difficult to make out, this hum, its specifics. Yes—that one. There. Hear it? Distant. Back. Back beyond the wall—that wall. Way back. Heating, I think. Yes, a boiler perhaps.

And *that* hum? Yes—pitched higher, nearer, in the room: my anglepoise lamp. I turn. The lamp illuminates one section of the lowest of three full bookshelves, casting light on only the letters R and S. Richardson to

Spry. Pelias, Tamas and Thiel are just possible to make out. Adams and Zizek are cast into darkness, like the letters of hell.

I use the lamp because the overhead strip-light is aggressive. I never use it, except when with a student or a colleague on a winter's afternoon and the subtle light of the lamp seems ill-advised and unnerving. An insinuation of uncomfortable intimacy.

I hold still. Or try to. I wish my body would find tranquillity, even if only for a moment. Allow itself to soothe and settle. Allow the currents to slow to just enough. Enough to keep moving, yes, to keep flowing, to keep alive; but this, what it does now, these days, and has been doing—this furious internal activity that wakes me with a start in the empty hours—is surely not entirely necessary.

Still. Wait. Listen. Heating hum. Check. Lighting hum. Check. And then—an interruption. Water. Pipes. Waste. Shit. Somewhere in the building there must be someone else. I thought I was alone.

In the department office yesterday, I knelt by a colleague's desk. (I kneel. It's a habit. To stand by her, or anyone, and talk from this height feels like standing over a refractory child I want to intimidate.) I knelt. She apologized. She didn't need to but she did. There's too much to do, she says. Whatever she does she's always behind. She will keep going and keep going, then take leave and on the first weekend get sick. Sick like the others who are not here because they have been made ill. I tell her please don't worry. I understand. And I know, as I say it, that understanding, such as it is, is impotent.

This is a sick building. Shit seeps from the pipes into the walls and through the floors, creeps through the cracks and the corners into our lives and into our bodies.

Still. Wait. Listen. The pick, drop, rub and scrape of construction outside the window. They start early, these men. The sweep of sand and cement. I can glimpse through my window pane, in the lamplight, scaffolding that spears skywards, leaving the tarmacked ground for shoes that scuff slow and quiet.

I seem only to sense, if at all, other bodies at this time of day. (Until the sound of waste through pipes.) Later, the rise of voices will bring their bodies to me through the crescent half-window one floor up.

I feel alone. The corridor is empty and dark. My neighbours' offices are empty and dark.

Breathe. Below my computer screen there is a card, blue and green, hand-drawn, a gift, a reminder for life, a reminder of life, a reminder of love. It speaks to me in black, irregular letters, the words: 'Don't forget to breathe'.

Shit Two

Room 4 at the counselling service on a Tuesday evening. I left my office with relief as the day darkened, and leaning into the cold easterly wind I walked the thirty minutes here through the green of The Meadows and along the busy rush-hour streets.

Karl undoes his suit jacket and looks up at me. He does not hesitate.

"I've hated this week. Nothing completed, nothing achieved. Just get up, go to work, and trudge through the daily bog. Through the crap. Stupid directives from the top, pointless meetings, people in the team falling out and one of them brings me her crumbling personal life, like she thinks I can resolve it. Sorting out her crap is not my job and I couldn't anyway, but what do I say? I do my best. Then I go home and it all starts again. My own crap all starts again. It's all still there. Everything I left when I walked out the door in the morning. It hasn't gone away. She's distant, and the boys are either out avoiding homework or home and sullen. And the TV is hopeless. More crap".

There are many possible responses I could make to this. Most would be harmless, at least; most would enable him, enable us, to take what he has said and work with it. I could ask him, for example, to say more about the specifics. I could enquire into the details of, say, his colleague's difficulties, wondering as I ask if they have echoes of his own; or the particulars of the interactions at home. Or I could just nod. Do the clichéd therapist thing. Go 'uh-huh'. I could do nothing. I could wait. Each of these might open something up, might prompt us to take this further, might *help*. But I don't do any of these. Instead, when he ends with "And the TV is hopeless. More crap", I say,

"That's a lot of crap".

And he raises his eyes again to meet mine and retorts, "You don't say".

He does not look away. He does not smile. There is no warmth in his sarcasm. It was the wrong moment for me to offer something light. I misread him. I misread it, the 'this', what was happening just now. Misread us. The way he looked, the tone of his voice. As a therapist intervention following a client making himself vulnerable, 'That's a lot of crap' did not rank amongst my best. "That was crass", I tell myself.

I half-smile. It is a weak move but it is an acknowledgement, if nothing else. After a few seconds he looks down, sits back and brings his hands together on his lap.

"It's too much. There's too much that can't be fixed out there. In all of it. Work and home. It's not what I thought it would be like".

"Yes, I can see that".

"Nor this, here".

"This isn't what you thought it would be like?"

"No. I didn't expect you to try to be funny".

"No".

"I didn't expect you to compound the crap with your own". Then adds, "If crap can be compounded".

SHIT THREE

Tuesday 24 February 2015, The Stand Comedy Club, York Place, Edinburgh

You've been queuing outside for half an hour along the street where the trams run; you're not the first in line, not the last, and you think you're early enough to get a seat and, if you're lucky, one with a table. It's blowing a gale and though your coat is thick the chill cuts you between hood and face and you don't chat to your mate; you just focus on trying to keep warm. The queue starts to move at last and you head down the twisting black metal stairs to the club. It's in the basement and it's low through the door and you feel you have to stoop though you don't. You owe your dues to the smiling member of staff with dyed red hair and it's just a fiver for tonight's show and you've ordered your tickets online so it's easy; you show your credit card and you're in. You pass another smiler on your left—she offers you a blue-yellow 'Bright Club' badge with a duck, which you take—and there's the bar on your right, but you go straight to the spare table you've spotted because the bar can wait; and you and your friend sit, shed coats and scarves and gloves and fold them under your chair and you see the candy on the tables and you know it's there to give you the sugar rush and make you more available for laughter and you think, 'god, how manipulative'.

An hour later you're on your third drink and the candy is all gone, what with you and your mate and the two girls in front of you with their backs to you whose drinks are on your table and who've been sharing the candy. There're no seats left anywhere and there's people behind you standing with their backs to the wall and their drinks on a shelf. There must be, you don't know, about sixty or seventy people in here and it's tight but you were never that good with numbers and especially not after a few drinks and a load of candy; and at last the lights dim and you know it's been coming, what with the five-minute warning they gave you, and the announcer with the big Scottish voice says "give a huge hand to your host for the evening—Jay Lafferty!" And she's not what you're expecting, she's young and cute, and in a couple of paces from the door to the right she's onto the stage; it's only about the size of your table and she makes the room fill with her voice through the mic and you already like her because she's relaxed and confident. She does the usual comedian thing of getting people to put up their hands and seeing who's from where and taking the piss out of the English and asking the idiots who sat at the front where they're from and imitating their accents, but she's kind and funny and everyone loves her. And she tells everyone about what 'Bright Club' is about (as if they didn't know): it's academics who are doing stand-up about their research and they're not professionals so don't give them a hard time, give her a hard time instead if you must, and if you do she'll fuck you over so don't bother trying.

Then she says to the guy at the front right at the end, ok so you start the clapping do you think you can do that, which makes him laugh, and then we'll go round the room, she says, as she sweeps her arm across, like a wave, like a surge of laughter, and we'll invite the first act on stage; and give him a warm welcome and I know you're going to love him and he's going to make you laugh and think at the same time, please welcome to the stage Jonathan Wyatt—'Counselling on a Scale of 1 to 5'!—sweep sweep sweep, clap clap clap, a quiet grumble building to a cheer, almost, as he comes out from the same door on the right. He's carrying a tea cup—why a tea cup?—and he shuffles past a man with the longest legs you've ever seen, then the woman behind the guy who started the clap (so to speak) then the guy himself who started the clap, then past Jay Lafferty who's stepped back to give him just enough room. Then he's on the stage, that tiny wooden stage, and he puts his cup on the table in front of him where there are two people looking up and watching for what he's going to be like, and then he puts his right hand on the mic stand and his left on the mic and he takes the mic from the stand and lifts the stand and reaches it behind so it's out of the way; and he's wearing a flowery blue button-down shirt, like a shirt you wear when you're trying to be someone who performs strand-up; and he's in jeans and converse boots that you can just make out between the heads of the two girls and the bushy-haired bloke and the bearded bald one right near the front.

And he looks like he might be a bit nervous but he's not shaking or anything and then he says: "This isn't part of my set but you might like to know that doing stand-up is a very good laxative".

***

'Ordinary affects'. That flow from and between bodies in rooms, in buildings, in spaces—with or of rooms, buildings, and spaces; affecting one another and generating intensities: human bodies, discursive bodies, material bodies, bodies of thought, bodies of water; sad bodies, troubled bodies. Laughing bodies, who might say, in that moment of abandon, that they couldn't give a shit about anything

Notes

183 A version of this chapter was first published as Wyatt, Jonathan, "Two Shits: A Connection of Some Kind". *Departures in Critical Qualitative Research* 5, no. 4: 43–47. That paper was in turn originally presented at the 11th International Congress of Qualitative Inquiry at the University of Illinois at Urbana-Champaign in May 2015, as part of a panel Alecia Jackson and I organized, in which we invited four others to join us in responding to Kathleen Stewart's *Ordinary Affects*.

184 Stewart, *Ordinary Affects*, 2007, 128.

Chapter 7

COUNSELLING ON A SCALE OF 1 TO 5

Edinburgh, February 2015

This chapter follows the previous one in telling the story of venturing on stage as a stand-up performer for the first time. My comedy set was based on my experience of being a counselling practitioner and researcher.

Sunday 15 February 2015

D-Day minus nine. I'm rehearsing my eight minutes in the back room at home, as I have been every day. I approach the centre of the room and mime taking the mic off the stand with my left hand whilst holding the stand still in my right, then placing the stand behind me to my right. I hold the hairbrush-mic just there, in my left hand, in the now-familiar position, out from under my chin, and look through the window outside over the courtyards. The script on the Kindle rests on the mantelpiece, ready if needed, and address my audience of cats, trees, walls and plants. I run through the text, and repeat. Over and over (including the mic removal manoeuvre at the top of the set), feeling the problem of getting words to stick in my body, for them to feel right, learning to trust the crafted script better than the words my body wishes to generate. Or, perhaps—yes—not yet trusting the text the body generates. Some of the written script wasn't right, I've realized as I speak it aloud, as I feel myself saying it: 'Counselling room',

I'd written; but 'consulting room' has better rhythm, with the emphasis on the second syllable. Who would have known? Most of the script seems to work, there on my own in front of my imaginary, but valued, audience. They break off from what they're doing to laugh at all the right moments.

There in the back room, in between taking calls from my sister about Mum's unhappiness now we have moved her to the new, cheaper home and how she is no longer eating, I've been worrying what it will be like if I miss phrases, how much it will disrupt my rhythm, how vulnerable I will feel if I lose it.

WEDNESDAY 18 FEBRUARY 2015

I walk up the steep hill to work, rehearsing as I go, muttering the words loud enough for me to hear and feel them but only just. There is a steady stream of people walking the opposite direction, probably to the large commercial buildings at the bottom of the hill. No one appears to think it strange, this man talking to himself, though some do glance. Perhaps they assume I am on my phone.

I pause the set as I stop to cross roads, which is prudent. I have learnt that I am unable to be vigilant about my safety at the same time as being fluent as a would-be comic. Do the professionals have this trouble, I wonder?

I call Mum from work. She went somewhere gorgeous today with my sister, but she can't remember where.

I call my brother, too, to catch up. We discuss playing golf when I'm down in a week's time. He reports on his visit to Mum, how he encountered Joyce, Mum's neighbour in the room next door, who used to be a paediatric surgeon, apparently the first British woman to be so. My brother and Joyce passed in the corridor as he was on his way to see Mum, and she stopped him to ask,

'Am I giving the lecture today?

'No', he replied, thinking quickly. 'I don't think so'.

'Are you giving it?', she pressed.

'No, I'm on next week'.

Joyce walked on, satisfied.

Thursday 19 February 2015

I rehearse some more, only this time with an audience of Dan, who organizes Bright Club in Edinburgh, plus an Andy and a Heather. An audience of three in a quiet room. It's like an audition. It's just me. The others performing on Tuesday have all done it before. There's a mic and a stand but no sound. I plough through the set, the words arriving when I need them to, more or less, just in time, Andy laughing twice but otherwise without discernible response, and I reach the end unscathed. The three of them offer positive, if muted, comment when I finish. I'm not sure if this indicates acceptance of the ordinary or something more optimistic.

Saturday 21 February 2015

Today we picked up a new car. It has cream leather heated seats.

We were on the point of driving it away and the guy remembers it's not taxed, so we have to get out and go back inside. While we're waiting I say to Tess,

"I'm a bit excited about my book".

"Which book?"

"The one I haven't written. But I've probably got to decide who I'm writing for. Counsellors or a wider audience. Or the usual crowd of 150". Then add, "Whom".

"Pardon?"

"*Whom* I'm writing for, not who. It's the accusative, 'for whom'. Dad would be twisting in his grave at 'who'. Except he was cremated. But still".

As the salesman returns towards us, I add: "Though 'whom' is clumsy. The language has moved on. Who I'm writing for. Sorry, Dad".

Tuesday 24 February 2015

4.30pm

Stand-up day. I have been at home, officially working and rehearsing but primarily panicking. My shoulders ache, and I forgot to go to my monthly clinical supervision meeting at 2.00pm. My supervisor texted me at 2.15pm to enquire, which was the first I realized.

I've shat four times.

In one run-through (of the stand-up script, that is), I forgot the main joke, the 'invisible' one. How did that happen? How come these words won't stick? How come they slip in and out of view at will?

In forty minutes, I will leave to walk up the hill to Queen Street and turn left to York Place and The Stand. A fifteen-minute walk at most, but I will find it difficult not to be there early. I'm restless. I don't know what to do with myself.

I'll go and rehearse again. 'Good evening, I'm Jonathan Wyatt'. That line I can remember.

8.00pm

I'm in the green room. I need to go again. I have a dry throat. I'm first on, in about 45 minutes' time, after the MC, Jay Lafferty, has warmed up the audience. In the rehearsal earlier to Dan and the handful of other performers I nearly lost my words at regular points. I hated it. Hated the flatness of the set. Waiting my turn I hadn't wanted to bother, but I did it and rushed through.

8.45pm

Time. Jay summons me on—'Please welcome to the stage—Jonathan Wyatt', cue cheering and clapping—let's go.[185] I open the door and walk. I'm carrying a cup of water, having not been able to find a glass. I pass Jay, who stands aside to let me pass and gives me a smile, and step onto the tiny stage, placing the cup on a table, after first—polite even *in extremis*—checking with those sat by it. I decide as I walk on that I'm going to just come clean. Be open. Tell it like it is. It crossed my mind earlier that I *might* but now, as I walk on, I think fuck it, I will. I take the mic off the stand, place the stand behind me—I have practised this move so often I am expert— and, holding the mic just below the chin, as trained and practised, I say,

> This isn't part of my set, but you might like to know that doing stand-up is a very good laxative.

What I actually mean, of course, is that *preparing for* stand-up, not *doing* it, not being here now, is a very good laxative. I'm surely flushed out by this point and the front row is safe. No one in the audience picks me up on this inaccuracy, thankfully. I get my first laugh, and I launch into the well-rehearsed script.

> Good evening. I'm Jonathan Wyatt. I'm a counsellor. A couns-ell-or. Not a councillor, counc-ill-or. I'm a therapist, not an elected member.

The audience is not your usual stand-up crowd. There are friends and colleagues of those of us performing, plus a few Bright Club devotees, and to Jay Lafferty's surprise in her banter before I go on stage, a hen party (a different one).[186] They're sitting at the back and aren't raucous or dressed in pink, and Lafferty never quite manages to get a coherent story out of them about why they've chosen a) a Tuesday night for a hen party and b) to come to Bright Club. It's probable they didn't realize. Whatever the audience's reason for attending, though, Lafferty's conversations with those present have ascertained that it is multi-national. So the point is this: does the term 'councillor' mean the same, or mean anything come to that, outside the UK? In the USA it's used to indicate that someone is a lawyer. Anyway, those opening lines seem not to fall flat, though I think this might be because of the phrase 'elected member'. In later performances of this set, I pause and add: 'Yes, that's my gratuitous knob joke. Elected member'. In case people don't get the innuendo; it would be a shame to let it go to waste, especially as it re-appears later in the set.

> I'm a counsellor, a therapist. I research what happens in the counselling room: the stories we bring there from our lives, how we talk about them there, and the stories we tell about what takes place there.

I read once that everything in stand-up should come in threes. Something about pace and rhythm, and unexpectedness. We're so used to thinking in binaries, either this or that, and a third can bring us up short. I think I over-do the threesomes rule, though. Here comes another; and another:

> So, it's mostly stories of pain, loss, and grief, sometimes hope, intimacy, love. Counselling is serious; and it isn't that funny.

I don't deal in numbers. I used to, when I worked for the NHS in a doctor's surgery. I had to fill in forms with patients, each time I saw them. With questions like, "On a scale of 1 to 5, how close to despair are you?" Where 5 is "despair, I laugh in your face" and 1 is "despair and me, we have a joint mortgage". We did those questionnaires at the end of each session. So that we could tell whether or not the counselling was working; how good a job I was doing. In seven minutes' time, I'll ask you that question.

The second time I did this set, in Newcastle, I didn't need to finish the sentence. "In seven minutes' time . . ." was sufficient. Maybe the difference was the delivery—more confident? Slower? A longer pause before the line? (See? Another set of three)—or maybe the different audience, the different space.

"No, I don't do numbers, I'm interested in the stories of counselling".

I pause. Then wait, searching. It's not that there's any laughter to hide behind as what I've just said hasn't elicited any. No, I'm waiting for the next line. I have no idea where I am in the script. I can't get hold of what comes next. This—losing my lines—is what I feared most and it hasn't taken long for it to happen. Nothing for it: I'll have to own up or the audience will wonder what's happening.

"I had a line there. . . .", I say, forlorn. This buys me a few seconds and a laugh and, as if by the magic of 'fessing up, there's the line, right where I left it—

Counselling is serious, not funny—and it's private. I can't just run from the consulting room to the laptop and write 'you'll never guess what she just told me. . .'

Not easy to talk or write about. I can change names, adjust the stories, wait a long time to publish, ask people's permission, but it's tricky.

So my research is also about the counsellor's stories, about what it's like to be a therapist, about what goes on inside us, how we understand what's taking place. That's easier to talk about, because at least it's about the counsellor not the client. The counsellor's stories, not the client's. My stories, not theirs.

So I don't think I'm breaching any ethical boundaries when I tell you that I once slept with a client.

I worked at the doctor's surgery on Wednesdays. I'd been to the States for a conference; flown back on the Monday. My last client of the day, Ellie, the middle of the session, about 5.45pm, twenty minutes in, two days after a long-haul flight and a very busy conference: she's telling me a story from her week, how she and her work colleague had fallen out over a stapler. I wake up when she's talking about a row with her partner over Silent Witness the night before. From the stapler to Silent Witness. I'd gone, drifted off. A few seconds perhaps, maybe more. A minute. However long it takes to get from office equipment to bad crime drama. She didn't notice, apparently. Or maybe she did but didn't care: maybe I was a better therapist when I was asleep. Or maybe she didn't have the heart to tell me. Or couldn't get angry with me: "Oi! Jonathan! Counsellor! Coun-sell-or! Wake the fuck up!"

So, that was Ellie, the client I slept with. She came back next time.

I fell asleep on another client too:

In the long gap between morning clients and afternoon clients I'd some-times walk home and have a little lie down.

It's going well. I'm not rushing. I'm enjoying it. I think, I can do this. What was I worrying about? Then I drop the mic. To be more accurate, I'm left holding the mic but the wire it's attached to flops to the floor. Just like that. I'd been holding the mic too tight, or too low, and pressed the release button with the edge of my little finger.

The immediate round of laughter at my pratfall is tinged with uncertainty and doubt. Doubt in me, doubt in this enterprise. To have to call on help would break the spell still further. I stoop down, pick up the recalcitrant wire, stand, fiddle, my hands shaking, and click. It's in. I have taken, maybe, thirty seconds, in all, and the audience has waited with a measure of concern and, I imagine, hope. Hope not in what will follow, not in expectation of the quality of the content, but simple hope that order will be restored, that everything will be okay.

I speak into the mic again, commenting, "So professional!", which elicits a wave of relief laughter ("he's managed to fix it and he's not been derailed")—and we're off again.

Where was I? Oh yes, having a lie-down at home in the afternoon. Once, though, I woke up at 4.30pm. 15 minutes late for my first afternoon client,

Darren. I leapt up and raced round to the surgery on my bike, like that kid in ET, to find Darren reading patiently in the waiting room. I grovelled, I tried to explain, I offered him an extra session. He came back next time too.

Serious, private, not funny: especially as the reason he'd come to see me was because he felt invisible.

It's problematic telling stories about clients, and telling clients' stories; and when you tell stories about being a counsellor you talk about clients. So another angle is to work with your own stories. Not others' stories of pain, loss and grief but your own.

I could talk about the episode in the Swiss hotel spa involving a cultural misunderstanding about dress code. There was the pain of my embarrassment, the severe loss of pride, and grief for my dignity. And a non-elected member.—

There's the knob joke call-back, one I remain proud of, but the audience doesn't laugh so I plough on—

But I can't tell you about that—I never even talked about it with my therapist. Therapists have therapists. It's a pyramid scheme. So I'll tell you an easier story, sleep-related. Long-term sleep. The moment my dad died. (So you've had politics and sex, and now you've got death.)[187]

This is a moment I've had concerns about. Whether the milieu of stand-up, or this specific stand-up event, with what has gone before and the sense and mood of the room, would 'hold' bringing the loss of my dad into the room. What would the audience do with it? How would they feel they were meant to respond? Later, a member of the audience told me he wondered where I was going with this but he told himself he just had to trust me.

We're gathered around his bed in the hospital. Mum, sister, brother, me. Sister Mary, too. She wasn't my sister, you understand—that's Nicola—she was some random nun.

We tell old, familiar stories. We tell him what a good dad he was. We tell him we'll look after Mum.

Sister Mary asks if she can pray. And my brother, Simon, prays too. God's victory over death, that kind of thing. (Now you've got religion.)

Dad breathes in, breathes out.

That's it. Gone.

Silence. Traffic outside the window; the sound of comings and goings in the corridor.

Stillness.

And then.

Dad sits up. Slow, steady, his upper body tilting from the bed. Not far, but further than you'd expect of a dead man. Cars crash; screams from the corridor. We leap from our seats. And my knee releases the neat little green button below the mattress.

As I'm saying this, I lift a straightened hand and forearm up and across my body, robotically, to indicate the raising, and sudden halting, of the bed. I haven't rehearsed this but intuitively realize, as I'm telling others this story, that the visual aid might help. It does. It's that gesture that seems to elicit the laughter, that seems to enable the audience to visualize this awful moment.

Serious, private, and on a scale of 1 to 5, pretty close to fucking hilarious.

I've been Jonathan Wyatt—counsellor. Thank you for listening.

11.05pm

Home. In the post-mortem excitement, Tess and our friend, Maggie, who has travelled up from Newcastle for this, say that the two funniest moments were when I forgot my lines and when I dropped the mic. When the unexpected happened. When it was out of control. When they, I, we all were taken by surprise.[188] Tess says she wonders why I needed to swear. It didn't sound right coming from me as I don't often swear. (Dan, at one rehearsal, advised, if in doubt, to swear. It always gets a laugh. It's a stand-up trope.)

2.05am

I can't sleep. Each time I close my eyes I'm on stage again. I'm still there, still in that darkened, crowded space; caught, taken. Surprise takes us. It comes upon us. Like on stage a few hours back; and like in that moment last week with not Karl but another client, Lillian, a moment that comes to me as I lie here: when she tells me how her teenage grand-daughter practised putting make-up on her during the week and Lillian says, "She

did a lovely job but, at my age, with my skin, I looked like a drag queen".
We laughed then and I laugh again here, in the still darkness.

Anything can happen.

NOTES

185 There's a film of this performance here: www.youtube.com/
watch?reload=9&v=yzkLUbgITwA

186 See Chapter 3.

187 There is a different version of this story, told for a different audience and
for a different purpose, in Wyatt, "A Gentle Going?", 2005.

188 See Chapter 4.

CHAPTER 8

"OUT HERE A MAN SETTLES HIS OWN PROBLEMS"

Learning From John Wayne[189]

Edinburgh, Spring 2014, Summer 2017, July 2018

This is a chapter about sons and fathers; or better, with creative-relational inquiry, it is a chapter about fathering: father as verb, as something-that-happens; father as continuous event. In the chapter I move between the experience of watching TV with my father, a stand-up performance by Scott Gibson about his father and the prospect (or not) of becoming a father himself and Karl bringing his father, and his being a father, into the counselling room. In relation to watching TV with my father, I focus on the figure of Tom Doniphon, the John Wayne character in the film "The Man Who Shot Liberty Valance", a "liminal hero"[190] living at the edge of town, as I consider the links between what my father and I watched together and how I learned, or did not learn, to find my way through my adolescent troubles.

WRITING, FRIDAY 13 JULY 2018

The story I told at The Stand in February 2015 of my father's dying has a different rendering in the first academic paper I wrote about him—about fathers, about loss—ten years before. I wonder about how he would have been with my taking his and our solemn, sacred, final moments and re-casting them as material for a seedy, alcohol-fuelled roomful occasion and a crowd of people looking to be entertained.

I keep writing about my father. He keeps appearing, he keeps becoming someone new, becoming *something* new, a colour changing shade. I miss him. I miss him in obvious moments, like at Christmas. I miss how we would look over the TV schedules together to plan the films we wanted to see. I miss the way he would sing the volume of Christmas in church and on people's porches as we did the carol singing rounds; and how, in my angry early twenties when I delayed returning home for Christmas as long as I could, he would tell me over the phone, in play but in sincerity, to come home sooner.

But it's not only at Christmas: some days, some moments, like leaving the apartment to climb the steps onto Dundas Street, I notice *not* seeing him. It's an instant of wishing his tall, upright profile into being caught against the clear sky as he waits for me by the black iron railings above.

I miss how he'd write funny lyrics to songs.

How he battled on, cheerful and obstinate and exasperating.

How he could speak in front a crowd, like at my sister's wedding, and make people laugh, and yet be so shy and reclusive.

I do not only miss him. I find him. He turns up, like when, as I write today in this month's favourite writing café near home, a child, sitting by me with her dad, laughs at the wiry-haired dog licking her hand. Is it that her delight reminds me of how my father could make children laugh? Or is it how he would often play with our dogs despite his espoused indifference? Or is it simply the life of that moment is somehow an echo of him-as-life?

After he died in 2003 I could not stop writing, paper after paper after paper, his stories turning and returning, demanding to be written as I continued to work at what loss means, at what loss does.[191] The urgency lessened after a time but he still appears as I write, like here, with Karl and with Scott Gibson, a reminder anew of what he invites: fathering as affective, affecting, continuing, creative-relational presence.[192]

THERAPY: KARL

Karl tells me he never knew his father. He told me this in an early session and we return to it.

"Never knew him?"

"No".

We've got here because we've been talking about his son. He's been telling me how his son won't spend time with him.

"I don't put pressure on him but I'd like him to feel he can be around me. He'll say good morning if I'm lucky. He's polite. If I'm lucky. But he

113

won't stay. He won't sit. He won't be around me. He doesn't *see* me. He's got to 15 and I've been dismissed. My services are no longer needed".

I check the clock, glancing down and across to my right. There's plenty of time, which I knew there was. Checking the time was checking out, for a moment. I can't catch why I needed to. Maybe it'll come to me later.

"He's sacked me. Much like she has, I suppose. Though she chose me at one point; he never did. When I look at him, which is mostly at his back as he leaves, I see me. I know, it's a cliché. But I wish I'd had me as a dad at his age. At least I *want* to know him. At least I *want* to be there. I am there. Whenever he needs me I'm there. Dad wasn't. Ever. He was physically there, well, at weekends, but he wouldn't talk to me. We'd sit for whole evenings. I'd be doing my homework or we'd be watching TV and he'd read the paper, half-watching. He wouldn't say much. He wouldn't ask me anything. He didn't show me he was interested even if he was. He worked away most weeks, the other side of the country, and came back at weekends".

He looks towards the window then back at me.

"I'm here, as much as I can be. I love the boy, and he won't be with me".

I didn't turn on the lamp at the back of the room, behind Karl, before we started, I notice. The early autumn light has faded and Karl is in shadow.

"I never knew Dad. All those years. Such a waste. I could do with him now. I could do with *me* now. A dad who's there. I guess he is and that's why I'm talking about him. He's just not here how I would have wanted him to be".

STAND-UP: SCOTT GIBSON

Scottish comedian Scott Gibson's father left Gibson and his brother when they were young. Old enough to remember, young enough not to understand; young enough to feel only the abandonment. Writing some weeks after seeing his show, *Like Father Like Son*,[193] it's difficult to remember what about this is funny, but it was. Overall, it was a delight—strong, poignant, surprising—but perhaps this section wasn't funny in itself. He makes the show's laughs about him, about being in his 30s with a partner who wants a baby; about how, therefore, he needs to lose weight. He's a big man and the room is hot, his sweat shimmering on him and on the floor. He isn't ready for children, he tells us, sounding playful, if frustrated and misunderstood. He's not ready to be a dad, and maybe he never will be, especially if being a dad means having to be like his brother, who Gibson paints as being earnest and indulgent with his children. He paints himself as impatient, uninterested and worse: hostile towards children. Gibson's father left not for the edges of their home town, Glasgow, but for the edges of Houston, Texas. A less than liminal dad.

Therapy: Karl

It's not only his boy, Karl says. He feels invisible to them all.

So, he's been walking. Walking the streets near his home alone, to see what happens; to not be the one who is left but be the one who leaves; to be the one who decides to be on his own, to take himself out to wander at the edges of his well-heeled, middle-class part of town, to work out what's possible, to search for something different through mundane, physical activity, through the "physicality of theorising", as St. Pierre might put it; to see if he can see himself; to see if he, anything, can settle.[194]

He stands at the front door and calls to anyone who's home—and who might be interested—that he's going out for one of his walks. "I'll be a while", he shouts, and waits. No response, mostly; though his wife sometimes calls back from her office, "OK. See you later".

Wherever he goes, everything feels familiar. He is never far from home. He walks as if he will never find something new; he knows the cracks in the pavements, anticipates the slabs that are loose and will rock and leave his shoes wet after rain. He logs with a droll smile the houses that have net curtains, finds pleasure in those whose gardens are neat, their patches of lawn trimmed, and notes the ones that construct gaudy Christmas decorations— Santa climbing the drainpipe, multi-coloured lights draped and flashing over outdoor fixtures, blown-up reindeer. He'd never have them himself, despite the kids' pleas when they were younger, but he likes to stand and watch them when they first appear; except those in place before December, which he resolutely ignores.

He tells me he lets the walk take control from the outset.

"When I'm on the pavement I turn whichever way draws me and I see where the walk leads. I go in the direction that feels right. It's a gesture to adventure".

"'A gesture to adventure'", he repeats. "See what I did there?"

"I do indeed".

"An enticement to excitement. A quest for zest. A run for fun".

Then he adds:

"No, that one doesn't work, does it? I don't run, for a start. Just amble. Peramble. Perambulate".

His playfulness wanders around the room, a curious and distracting child. I take us back to where he was. "You say it's all familiar, that you know every pavement slab, every garden, every tasteless Christmas house-owner. So, how does that feel like zest and excitement. Tell me more about the adventure".

He looks down at his hands, turning them over, this way and that. Like he's looking for something. I feel my invitation has been too abrupt, too intrusive, too dull.

Karl seems stalled but he lifts up his head and continues, despite my clumsiness. "I never know what will catch me that time", stabbing a finger onto the other palm for emphasis, "on that particular walk. I don't know what window, what tree, whose front door. That's where the adventure is, I suppose. But I agree, it's not adventure, and the rest of it is dull. I know. I know. I was being ironic".

He's sad. Deflated. His voice diminished.

"Sometimes I walk past houses the kids used to go and play in when they were small, the houses of friends they made at primary; and I have to stop and look, just look. I never know whose it will be until I pass and remember".

He adds, "I don't loiter suspiciously, you know. And this isn't every time I go out. You don't need to have the conversation with me about people being at risk. You don't need to tell me you might have to talk to the authorities but you'd prefer it if I did so myself".

I laugh, surprised. "Point taken. That wasn't what I was thinking".

At most of the houses he doesn't loiter outside his kids have long since lost touch with their friends, interests diverging or secondary school destinations different. He stops, he says, and wants to knock on the doors and catch up. Find out where those small kids are now, how they're turning out, what they're doing, how their school lives have been, how they are with their parents. He wants to talk to the parents too, whichever parents might still live there. He finds himself speculating about what's changed on that score. Who's still together, who's been replaced, which dad—as it usually is, he tells me wearily—has lost touch with their kids.

For a time, back then, some of those parents felt like his friends too, and Shell's. Couple-friends. People they'd have barbecues with in the summer so the kids could play together. Everyone would behave as if they liked each other. Some he did like, it's true, but some he didn't, and he knew it at the time.

"The company was welcome, but sometimes it was forced. Having conversations about water conservation with one environmental engineer dad, I remember. We stood for an age, bottles of beer in our hands. It was an effort. I know water conservation is important but I didn't want to get into it on a Sunday lunchtime. He was a nice guy though and it was all respite from the relentlessness of the kids. They had their friends to mess around with and left us alone for a while. Love them though I did. Do".

He never does approach the front doors. Through the gaps in curtains he catches fleeting sight of large teenaged boy-feet resting on the arm of a sofa, or the passing head of a dad looking purposeful and stern, or the stillness of a mum with hands on hips, or perhaps a hug exchanged between Mum and daughter. It would seem too weird to intrude on these domestic events, ones much like his own he imagines, and he knows they wouldn't welcome being intruded upon by someone who seems familiar but who they couldn't place. It would be awkward and embarrassing.

So he leaves them behind, taking his wistfulness with him, the textures different each time, and walks on. He wanders around the estates of the middle-class suburban 1930s houses, all much like his own; he traces the routes his sense of adventure takes him, and, after ten, twenty, thirty, sixty minutes, he twists the Yale key in the wooden front door and shouts, "I'm home", and no one answers. No problems have been settled.

WATCHING JOHN WAYNE

Before first writing the conference paper that became this chapter I did not know for sure that I ever saw *The Man Who Shot Liberty Valance*,[195] where John Wayne's maverick liminal hero, Tom Doniphon, lives at the edges of society, between 'good' and 'bad', between 'tough' and 'gentle'. A man with a mysterious, painful past, he tells James Stewart's idealistic lawyer, Ransom Stoddard, that "out here a man settles his own problems". I may have seen it. I have now.

If I had watched that film it would have been with my father one week-day evening, probably around 7pm, when Westerns were shown on TV during the 1970s. I would be about thirteen. Fourteen, maybe. At home from boarding school for the holidays. Dad would be sitting on the floor of my parents' bedroom. I would be lying on their bed. He would be busy, dealing with bills and correspondence, everything laid out in neat piles and ordered rows on the three-foot by two-foot patch of carpet that served as his desk. He had his own study just off the bedroom with a broad, solid wooden desk but this is where he would attend to what needed doing: with us, legs crossed on the floor and we on the bed. Maybe it would be him and me, just the two of us, or perhaps my brother and sister too, the three of us lying side by side across the bed. My mother might be there, watching and not watching. She would have preferred something on another channel, the travel documentary or the one on Richard III. She would have complained, perhaps, but lightly, or so I took it to be at the time. She was there because we were there.

Dad and I—and whoever, but I remember it as Dad and me, such memory, after Derrida, "constituted by the labours of mourning"[196]—would watch Westerns. And James Bond. Especially Sean Connery, of course. As the years progressed, our broadening tastes would come to include Kojak, Starsky and Hutch, Columbo, Cagney and Lacey, Charlie's Angels or their British equivalents The Sweeney and The Professionals. These Brit shows portrayed hard men in hard, downtrodden, downbeat towns, cops working in pairs: gruff, violent, snarling, indicative of angry 1970s and 1980s UK.

On Saturday afternoons, for Dad and me it would be the wrestling. Always at 4.00pm. Always on ITV. The British version of wrestling. Black and white, in rundown halls in downtrodden, downbeat English towns. Wrestlers like the heels—the baddies—Big Daddy and Giant Haystacks, against the blue-eyes—goodies—Kendo Nagasaki and Mick McManus. Or maybe Mick McManus was a heel. Big Daddy was a heel for a time and turned himself into a blue-eye.

But I digress. Or perhaps I don't. Goodies and baddies. This is the world my father and I inhabited when we watched whatever it was we watched. There were good guys and bad guys. The good-looking, well-muscled, strong but ethical wrestlers against the ugly, fat, hirsute, rule-breaking wrestlers. The flawed but decent cops, Starsky, Hutch, et al., against the murderous baddies. In the Brit versions, this distinction was more blurred—the cops themselves worked on the edge of both the law and of what might count as 'good', but we rooted for them and their subversive, anti-establishment, get-the-baddies-at-all-costs, ends-justify-the-means ethical position. Though I doubt they considered themselves as having ethical positions.

Stand-Up: Scott Gibson

We're at the end of a row where we can stretch out our legs, in an upstairs hall in the university's student association building amongst a near-full crowd. The room doesn't feel like a stand-up venue. With its square shape, its stark wooden floors, the dull walls and the rows of chairs, it's more like being at a school assembly, with an unlikely and intimidating head teacher giving us our weekly moral encouragement.

Gibson paces. I like him, I think. Or I keep telling myself I do. I'm afraid of him. He looks like he could be one of those wrestlers my dad and I watched, all bulk and beard, and he inhabits his body to the full, pacing and raging, sharp-eyed and sharp-tongued, spitting out the words as he rants about not wanting to diet or how he'd hate having to be patient if he were a dad. I sit with my friend, Marc, out of Gibson's eye line to the side a few rows back. But Gibson is not one of those performers who takes on the audience. We're not his target, and nor is his dad, not even when he gets into the material about how his dad stopped calling from the States or when Gibson, at 14, went over to visit and his dad gave so little time to him. Not even when he reports how his dad returned to Glasgow a couple of years ago, apparently to look after Gibson's grandfather and later told Gibson his liver was failing.

I have empty seats to my right and can turn to stretch out my legs towards the main body of the audience. We're laughing but it's not clear why. It's something about him, how he can be fierce and angry and show the pain at their source. It's like we see it but he doesn't, though we know he must, and that's his skill. I look round at the audience. Half full, perhaps more. Mostly men and mostly white, I notice.

Watching John Wayne

Black characters didn't figure often in the TV my dad and I watched. And if they did, they were the light relief. The grass, Huggy Bear, and his loping

119

nonchalance. In the man-cop shows, the women were pretty and bland. In the woman-cop shows things were more complicated. Pretty, bland and tough in Charlie's Angels. More ordinary and grittier in Cagney and Lacey.

And the Westerns—those I remember, or the aspects of those I remember— seemed always to have the equivalent of wrestling's blue-eyes and heels, goodies and baddies. The heroes were strong, rugged men protecting good but ineffectual men, children and pretty, skirted women from ruthless, mean men. Horses, cattle and dogs played their bit parts, all set amongst a pitiless, mean landscape and its downbeat, downtrodden, rundown towns. Sometimes, most times, the baddies were the 'redskins', 'Indians', who were silent, stealthy assassins or unruly hordes on horse-back. Surrounding and circling waggons containing terrified, blameless (white) citizens, the war-painted, bare-torso-ed warriors—the Sioux, the Commanchees—issued their shrill war-cries and swept in in a seemingly chaotic stream, to kill and scalp their victims with impassive delight. Late, but not too late for the characters that mattered, across the hills would come the cavalry or its equivalent, led by Custer or some other white, handsome hero.

I may be mis-remembering. But, anyway, I was oblivious at the time to the political assumptions I was buying into. I watched for the escape, because it was home not boarding school; because I could, because there was TV at home and no TV at school. And no Dad. Because, for those few weeks of the school holidays I could sit and watch TV with my father and the world would be simple and life's problems would be resolved within 90 minutes. I watched, wanting to be more like troubled, tragic outsider, Doni-phon, than hapless, though successful, establishment blue-eye Stoddard. I watched alongside my strong, good, oblivious father, yearning for John Wayne to come back to school and help me like he helped Stoddard. There, by my dad, I could try to find the Tom Doniphon in me who could settle his own problems. But I never could, and Doniphon was wrong, and should have known he was wrong, given it was he who came to Stoddard's aid.

When the Liberty Valances amongst my peers took pot shots at my ear-nest Stoddard-esque character, there was no Doniphon, no John Wayne, in the shadows firing them down for me. Out there a boy couldn't settle his own problems, or this boy couldn't. I just couldn't. I tried. I did what Stoddard did: I went out to face them. I went out to face them each day but I couldn't face them down, not alone. I kept trying, enlisting help from those who could have helped but didn't, or couldn't; kept trying until, in the end, I slipped out to the edges of town. With no Doniphon in the shadows covering my back, it was all that was left to do.

But then, there had been no Doniphon either for the boys I had, in my time, ruthlessly and systematically taken it out on; until one in particular, Turner (we never used first names), disappeared, not returning to school after the summer break.

Therapy: Karl and After Karl

After Karl, after the notes that need writing, after saying the usual cheerful goodbyes to my fellow Tuesday counsellors, I leave the building soon after 9.00pm and walk to the bus stop. It's a ten-minute wait. I check my phone. A message from home and one from Holly, just finishing hockey practice. A look at the football scores. It's a European night. Hopefully City are winning and Chelsea losing, but when I look I see that they're both still nil-nil. It's cold. I pull my coat tight around me. No one else is waiting. The bus turns the corner and I have my choice of seats. Tuesday in late autumn and everyone is at home.

I sit near a window, stretch out and close my eyes. I walk with Karl. I walk as I sit. I walk in my smart, black shoes, pacing the pavements, one step in front of another, until something arrests me. Life. Envy. Loss. All of those, perhaps. I know what he means. When it's dusk and curtains aren't yet drawn, it's possible to see into people's lives for a moment as you pass. You wonder if the middle-aged woman watching the news, or the young man ironing his white shirt, or the friends with wine in their hands, are happy. Happier than you.

The bus turns a corner and I'm thrown to my left, my head touching the window. I'm surprised and open my eyes. I feel alone. I am alone. We stop and two women alight, talking. They're still wearing blue aprons. Nursing assistants, perhaps, from one of the care homes nearby. They sit two rows in front of me and continue talking. It seems to be about one of their adult children who's found new work away from the city. I close my eyes again. I think of Joe in Seoul. He has been away so long.

Stand-Up: Scott Gibson

Scott Gibson travelled to Manchester for a gig the weekend his dad was due to move from living with Gibson's grandfather into his own flat.

"Don't, Dad. Leave it till I'm back. You shouldn't do the move on your own. You need help with it". In Manchester, he got the call next day: his dad had been carrying gear to the van and had collapsed.

After weeks of recovery, his dad moved from hospital to live with Gibson, with Gibson as his *de facto* carer. Gibson describes walking out of his bedroom into the corridor to find his dad's shit on the floor.

His dad is now in a home, which Gibson visits when he can.

He watches his father, surrounded by much older people, shrinking into a body that no longer seems to resemble the father who left over 20 years ago. Sees his father leaving, again. Leaving differently, finally. He speculates what stories his father will have to tell from wherever he's going. Gibson sounds like he wants this, wants contact with his father even as he reminds us that because of their relationship he doubts his own potential as a father.

As his show ends, Gibson, alone on stage, seems smaller, though his tone is cheery and he leaves with a quip about never becoming a dad. Marc and I leave. I see the poster outside the room that boasts quotes about the show's hilarity. I wonder how and why the poster omits to speak of the show's sadness, anger or even its vitality. Maybe none of those would be a good sell for a stand-up gig.

Writing, Friday 13 July 2018

In my writing-café this morning I had found a corner table to write the beginning of this chapter, a high table with only stools to perch on. I wasn't comfortable, but I stayed as long as I needed to find a way to begin.

The café was quiet for a Friday and the two baristas nearby were chatting in English about the football, the World Cup that's drawing to a close this weekend. Neither was English and they made no mention of England's valiant elimination on Tuesday. My melancholy is passing but I have felt alone with my sense of loss here in Scotland, where some want only humiliation for England but most are indifferent. I assumed both the baristas' countries had either also been knocked out or had not made it to Russia as neither sounded French or Croatian, but either way they both sounded cheerful and engrossed. Meanwhile, as I sat, writing and listening, the little girl left with her dad, waving goodbye to her dog friend, who had wanted to follow but couldn't, restrained by its lead looped around the table leg.

I am at my desk back home now; it's early afternoon, the long, balmy, dry spell being broken by welcome light rain that I can hear on the verdant foliage outside the open window. These fathers, these fathering presences: Karl and Karl's father, Gibson and Gibson's father, me and mine. They stream through and around and with me now. They, we, feel vivid and vibrant; and elusive. Ghosts. Not Doniphon shadows, but ghostly matterings, with all "their ambiguities, [their] complexities of power and personhood, [their] violence and the hope".[197] Assemblages, events; somethings-that-happen-and-continue-to-happen.

NOTES

189 An earlier, much shorter, version of this chapter was published as Wyatt, Jonathan, "Out Here a Man Settles His Own Problems": Learning from John Wayne. *International Review of Qualitative Research* 8, no. 3: 280–282, and in turn before that as a contribution to a panel on Westerns, one of an annual series curated by Bryant Alexander, at the 2014 International Congress of Qualitative Inquiry.

190 Poulos, "The Liminal Hero", 2012.

191 Wyatt, "A Gentle Going?", 2005; Wyatt, "Psychic Distance", 2006; Wyatt, "No Longer Loss", 2008; Wyatt, "What Kind of Mourning?", 2010; Wyatt, "Fathers, Sons, Loss", 2012.

192 Ron Pelias writes: "[My father] is a centre of my affective life. I am always writing him, even at times when I do not recognise that I am doing so. He is always present, always watching, as I am watching him". Pelias, *A Methodology of the Heart*, 2004, 74.

193 24 August 2017, Gilded Balloon and Dead Sheep Comedy.

194 St. Pierre, "Nomadic Inquiry", 2000, 267.

195 Ford, *The Man Who Shot Liberty Valance*, 1962.

196 Krell, *The Purest of Bastards*, 2000, 19.

197 Gordon, *Ghostly Matters*, 2008.

INTERVAL

Towards Creative-Relational Inquiry (2): The Problem and Promise of the Personal

Take it to heart, Massumi writes. There is a 'heart' to creative-relational inquiry, I asserted in the first Interval: what we might call a personal. I work further at this claim here.

The chapters of Part 2 of this book were, one might say, 'personal'. I have written of my father, of this man sitting on the floor while we watch TV. I have told the story of telling the story of his passing. I have spoken of my brother, my sister, my mother. I have written of Karl and his father, a shadow, a silhouette, who remains with him still and of how he was with us as we talked. I talked about Karl and his boy, who seems to Karl to be turning away from him, rendering Karl invisible, in turn, despite his efforts and heartfelt intent to be available to his son. Then there was Scott Gibson, a force on a stage, his loss and rage and doubt coursing through the mid-afternoon audience. I brought the personal—and the relational, in a humanist sense—onto the page. They are my stories, too, stories about 'me' and my relationships with human others. They are personal. They use personal pronouns ('I', 'you', 'we', etc.).

The theoretical framing(s) I embrace through this book—Deleuze and Guattari, new materialism, affect theory—offer a challenge to the personal. They challenge the personal's assumed human-centeredness. They argue— variously—against the personal's implicit assumptions of the unitary, essentialist, humanist subject, which can no longer hold in a flattened, immanent ontology, where "we are part *of* the world in its ongoing intra-activity [. . .] we are part of that nature we seek to understand".[198]

As St Pierre writes concerning the future of qualitative research in light of such theories, the personal (as commonly understood) is one of many shibboleths we will need to find a way to let go of as we re-imagine qualitative inquiry:

> [This future] will not be easy for those of us who have been well trained in qualitative methodology. What concepts from the old empiricism will we want to hang on to? Research designs like 'case study' and 'autoethnography' ('I' after 'I' after 'I')? Methods of data collection like 'interviews' and 'observations' ('I' after 'I' after 'I')? Concepts like 'data' (meaningful words in interview transcripts and field notes) and methods of data analysis like 'coding data' and 'cross-case analysis' (positivist practices)? Perhaps we cannot give up rich thick description, the language that represents the real. But the order-words of the old methodology will surely keep us stuck in the old ontology. This ontological turn of the new empiricism will require a great deal from us, because there are no textbooks, handbooks, workshops, or university research methods courses that tell us how to begin and then what to do next.[199]

In this account the 'I' (and other personal pronouns) is a writing habit we (sic) need to shed, a tired and, worse, under-theorized, trope that it is time we abandoned alongside the other taken-for-granted, received and unquestioned wisdoms of what elsewhere St. Pierre terms "conventional qualitative inquiry".[200]

Others working with and within these theoretical fields echo St. Pierre's challenge to the personal: Jackson and Mazzei critique autoethnography[201] for its reliance upon the apparent coherence of the narrator's personal account of unproblematic access to 'experience', calling instead for "a deconstruction of how the researchers' experiences constrain and limit what they can know and how they represent their participants or even their own social worlds".[202] They are not appealing for an abandonment of the personal, it is true, but they are arguing for a personal that is at least problematized. De Freitas and Paton, invoking Lacan, Derrida and de Man, call attention to how writing 'the self' is inherently contradictory and erasing: "Autobiographical acts . . . are acts of ellipsis and erasure as much as they are acts of constitution".[203] Writing the self, they suggest, without conveying, even if only at times, the assumption of the bounded, humanist self, is well-nigh impossible.

As one flow in our work, Ken Gale and I likewise have also been working with the challenge to the personal that comes with embracing, to use St. Pierre's term above, the "ontological turn". Ken and I have been writing together since 2005, writing collaboratively with each other and with others (including, throughout, with Deleuze) into the possibilities opened by collaborative writing-as-inquiry into thinking about and theorizing subjectivity. (I am writing with Ken still, now, as I write this apparently sole-authored book. I will always write with Ken.[204])

Ken and I have troubled and extended the bounded, autonomous individual subject-who-knows arguably implicit, for example, in the 'auto' of autoethnography, by proposing the concept of assemblage/ethnography,[205] the subject as Deleuzoguattarian assemblage, and we have continued to push at where this might lead us, at how to write.[206] We don't always agree and our discussions are often passionate. In one exchange, Ken, invoking Borges' nounless world of Tlon,[207] has been arguing for a move away from 'nouning' and for leaving personal pronouns aside. He writes,

> [My] writing above is full of scabs; there is a profusion of 'I's', 'we's', 'me's' and so on. This writing is about infection: it is infected. Its sores are virulent; they seep all over the page, messing with its honest intent, staining its integrity with the irrevocability of their creeping presence.[208]

In our discussion to this point, I have been full of resistance to this. Our exchanges have gone back and forth as we have been working at it. Here, I respond to Ken:

> I have been writing this in my sleep these last two nights; when its intensities have become too much, the writing has been waking me. I turn and turn, and it will not let me go. I am beginning this at work in my office, with an indecisive low sun of late autumn mid-afternoon causing me to raise and lower my blinds every few minutes, and I both welcome and am irritated by it.
>
> A question has come into view, one that seems to be (at) the heart of this chapter, this assemblage/ethnography; even, perhaps, at the heart of autoethnography in general. I will try to frame it:

To what extent can writers—people?—we?—lay claim to singularity? In our writing, in our lives.

No, that's not right. Well, yes, maybe, but perhaps this is better:

To what extent can we—do we, inevitably—create such singularity through writing; in writing between us; in this assemblage of (the verbs) Ken and Jonathan.

No, that's still not right. Yes, maybe it is; but there's more:

To what extent is it our political, ethical charge that we do so? That we must, because there is so much at stake.

You see, what, I think, is keeping me awake is how much these questions matter (in that word's various meanings) to me, to us, to the work. Here are today's answers to them:

However inadequate, however provisional, however misleading, we can and we must claim the possibility of singularity; we can and must aspire to, and work at, creating such singularity through writing. It is indeed our political and ethical charge. We have to. When I talk about singularity I am talking here of the 'singular existant' of Nancy,[209] which 'may be singular plural or something else entirely, outside of the order of the calculable';[210] a "haunted subject, haunted by what comes after it just as much as by what comes 'before', it can never be fully present to itself".[211]

I am with Rosi Braidotti in viewing the subject as:

> "an entity fully immersed in the process of becoming, in productive relations of power, knowledge, and desire. This implies a positive vision of the subject as an affective, productive and dynamic structure".[212]

You see, I am with her in seeing the subject as a—fluid, open, permeable—'structure', an 'entity' and, the term she invokes later, 'a figuration'.[213] I am with her in a call to the notion of 'bodily materialism', the "embodied or enfleshed subject",[214] one that is always "emerging out of a process of becoming."[215] With her in seeing nomadism as about "becoming situated, speaking from somewhere specific and hence well aware of and accountable for particular locations".[216]

I am with Kottman, talking of Cavarero, when he describes how she:

> "insists that the self is narratable and not narrated. It is an existence that has not been reduced to an essence, a 'who' that has not been distilled into the 'what'. In short, for Cavarero, it is the unique,

individual existent—who is in constitutive relation with other exis-
tents, and who is not yet, or no longer, a subject—who takes 'priority',
so to speak".[217]

This is why I am calling you, calling us, to stories in (this) assemblage/
ethnography. Cavarero, like you, like me, is against categorisation, simplistic representation, fixity, all of these, but argues that 'narration reveals
the finite in its fragile uniqueness, and sings its glory'.[218] This is why I keep
coming back to you to tell stories—not ones that are simplistic and unitary
but ones that provide, create, something of the embodied, the embedded,
the particular. You. Us. Me: writing this here, troubled, disturbed, angry,
passionate, joyful.

You see, in part I am fuelled by how I experience you. The theory you
espouse is not how I find you (the verb), today, in this moment. I don't
believe you want to live without calling on 'Reuben', 'Phoebe', 'Katie' and
those intimate others in your life; I don't believe that you want to live without telling me—you, others—how intense was yesterday's swim, say, your
body's immersion in the waves, its pull against the currents, the thrill; you
will always call on your trip to the US in 1989. You talk about yourself and
your life, your histories and your futures, your longings and desires, your
fears and anxieties—and so you should. You must. Dosse talks of Deleuze
and Guattari's 'intersecting lives', and tells their complex, nuanced, incomplete stories.[219] You and I joke about Deleuze's dodgy hair; we speak of their
differences, and of Guattari's work at La Borde and of his influence upon
their collaborative work.

Intensities, haecceities, flows, assemblages, all. I can't quite believe you
would want to live in Borges' world, though I know it only from what you
have told me. I wouldn't want to.

I am [. . .] with Gannon in arguing for "a relational autoethnographic
[or, rather, assemblage/ethnographic] subjectivity, a self that is contingent on
the recognition of others, and a self who finds voice through that relation".[220] By 'self', I mean that which is—echoing you above—a "contingent
result of an ongoing process".[221]

We must hold onto the possibility of the personal, the personal pronoun,
the person, the relational. There are politics at stake here. For Braidotti,
memory and narrative are crucially linked to "practices of accountability
(for one's embodied and embedded locations) as a relational, collective
activity of undoing power differentials".[222] To not do so is disabling and

nihilistic: "The world without me, the-world-without-us... (is) the folk tale of the end";[223] and it is to abdicate responsibility; to fall, ironically, into self-referential indulgence.

This is where I will end today. I will not place the personal pronoun in inverted commas.

It's now Saturday morning. I'm at home. Tess has gone out for a day with her fellow students and tutors on the Masters programme she is so much in love with. You have sent me more writing that I have glanced at but now want to engage with fully. You have sent me an email about your antics last night, and about how much you enjoy Friday nights, which I do too—better than Saturdays by far, I agree. Now I must wrest myself from this writing and take in some air. And get coffee.[224]

I find, now, some years later, I can only continue to make this bid for the personal within creative-relational inquiry. I find I cannot but think and write with the personal, including here throughout this book. I use the personal pronoun. I tell personal stories: stories about my mother, father, family; stories others—mostly, stand-up performers—tell of people in their lives; and stories of the people (though it is mostly just the one, Karl) I see in my clinical work as a therapist. I am drawn to such stories. They need telling.[225] Creative-relational inquiry calls for relating, in this sense too, for the narrating of stories. "Stories, like paths, relate in two senses: they recount and they connect".[226]

It may be my insistence on the personal is wanting both to have my theoretical cake and eat it. Maybe it is to do with the inevitable grammatical and syntactical traps of writing, or writing in English at least. It may be, as St. Pierre says, it is to do with attachment to old, entrenched ontological habits.[227] And/or it may be because of an aversion to impersonality, as Melissa Orlie argues, "a defence against experiencing or acknowledging the impersonal forces that compose us".[228]

These attributions may be fair, but I would argue—or maybe only hope—they are not all of the story. The personal—the I, you, me, s/he, they—of this book draws its voices from the "collective assemblage",[229] an assemblage I am mostly unconscious of; and writing, as Deleuze and Guattari argue, is a process of allowing such voices to emerge, enabling the collective to "give way" to the personal[230]—for a moment, tentatively, provisionally.[231] In so doing, creative-relational inquiry refers not to the fixed, centred, bounded, unitary, denominative subject but to something like Caverero's *unique existent*, about which I wrote to Ken.[232]

Cavarero's concept concerns 'who' not 'what'. The unique existent, Cavarero writes, like the shape-shifting *daimon* of Greek myth, is always behind our backs, needing the other's recognition and therefore always vulnerable, always incomplete. It is characterized by desire, she says, and in particular the desire for narration by the other: "The story . . . has at its centre an unstable and insubstantial unity, longed for by a desire that evokes a figure—or rather, the unmasterable design—of a life whose story only others can recount".[233]

This, then, may be the 'personal' of creative-relational inquiry: never, in fact, about a *person*, in that term's common-sense, humanist meanings, but nevertheless always about a (dynamic, hyphenated) *you*.[234]

NOTES

198 Barad, "Posthumanist Performativity", 2003, 828.

199 St. Pierre, "Deleuze and Guattari's Language for New Empirical Inquiry", 2017, 1087.

200 St Pierre, "Decentering Voice in Qualitative Inquiry", 2008, 332.

201 See note 63, Chapter 3, Always More. Autoethnography is "an autobiographical genre of writing and research that displays multiple layers of consciousness, connecting the personal to the cultural". Ellis and Bochner, "Autoethnography, Personal Narrative, Reflexivity", 2000, 739.

202 Jackson and Mazzei, "Experience and 'I' In Autoethnography", 2008, 309.

203 de Freitas and Paton, "(De)Facing the Self: Poststructural Disruptions of the Autoethnographic Text", 2009, 498.

204 As I have claimed earlier, we are always writing with others: Pineau, "Haunted by Ghosts", 2012; Speedy, "Collaborative Writing and Ethical Know-how", 2012.

205 e.g. Wyatt and Gale, "Getting Out of Selves", 2013; Gale and Wyatt, "Assemblage/Ethnography", 2013.

206 See Gale and Wyatt, "Working at the Wonder", 2017; Wyatt and Gale, "Writing to it", 2018.

207 Borges, *Labyrinths*, 1971.

208 Gale and Wyatt, "Assemblage/Ethnography", 2013, 141.

209 Nancy, *Being Singular Plural*, 2000.

210 Callus and Herbrechter, "Introduction", 2012, 246.

211 Callus and Herbechter, 246.

212 Braidotti, *Nomadic Subjects*, 2011, 17.

213 Brians, "The 'Virtual' Body", 2011.

214 Braidotti, *Nomadic Subjects*, 2011, 15.

215 Brians, "The 'Virtual' Body", 2011, 133.

216 Braidotti, *Nomadic Subjects*, 2011.

217 Kottman, in Cavarero, *Relating Narratives*, 2000, xii.

218 Cavarero, 3.

219 Dosse, *Intersecting Lives*, 2010.

220 Gannon, "Sketching Subjectivities", 2013, 228.

221 Brians, "The Virtual Body", 2011, 132.

222 Braidotti, "Nomadism", 2010, 410. See also Stephanie Springgay and Sarah Truman's argument for posthuman theoretically informed work to take account of its politics. In their book, *Walking Methodologies*, concerning the theorizing and practice of 'walking-with', they state: "Walking-with is explicit about political positions and situated knowledges. . . . Walking-with is accountable. Walking-with is a form of solidarity, unlearning, and critical engagement with situated knowledges. Walking-with demands that we forgo universal claims about how humans and non-humans experience walking, and consider more-than-human ethics and politics of the material intra-actions of walking research". Springgay and Truman, *Walking Methodologies*, 2018, Routledge, 11.

223 Callus and Herbrechter, "Introduction", 2012

224 Gale and Wyatt, "Assemblage/Ethnography", 2013, 148–150.

225 I once wrote: "How can a poststructuralist writing about personal experience be anything but ironic, and how can a therapist write about their clients ironically?" Wyatt, "Ash Wednesdays", 2013, 132.

226 MacFarlane, *The Old Ways*, 2012, 105.

227 St. Pierre, "Deleuze and Guattari's Language", 2017.

228 Orlie, "Impersonal Matter", 2010, 120.

229 Deleuze and Guattari, *A Thousand Plateaus*, 2004, 93.

230 Manning, *Always More Than One*, 2013, 28. See also Murray, "When Dust Gets in Your Eye", 2017.

231 I note how the Deleuzoguattrian "collective assemblage" is echoed by Patrica Clough in her notion of the 'user unconscious', and how this in turn calls for a 'thickening' of this discussion of the personal. Clough cites Wendy Hui Kyong Chun's concept of the 'YOU', the networked subject that lives in social media (Chun, *Updating to Remain the Same*, 2016). As with Deleuze, Manning and others cited here, this leads also to a reconsidering of common-sense humanist understandings of the boundaries of the body. Clough writes: "I would propose that digital media and computational technologies may well be eliciting the human user's thing-self, giving shape to what I am calling the user unconscious in order to point to the activity of the unconscious in relationship to the collapse into the YOU, of the I and the cloud of digital traces, including the data of a worldly sensibility. These, no matter how disavowed, are becoming an intimate part of the I, evoking a thing-self that opens the unconscious both to the liveliness of other-than-human actants and to the reformulation of embodiment in the YOU. That is to say, the YOU refers to that part of the I that is not humanly embodied, not so much a digital disembodiment, but an other-than-human embodiment. The I is not

simply humanly embodied and, as such, is not one with the organism. Embodiment cannot be contained within the organic skin". Clough, *The User Unconscious*, 2018, loc. 476–482, Kindle.

232 Cavarero, *Relating Narratives*, 2002.

233 Cavarero, 63.

234 Cavarero. There is a discussion to be had, for another day, about the distinctions and connections between Cavarero's *you* and Chun's YOU.

Part 3

Reframings[235]

---

235 Therapy, stand-up and writing each can enable difference to emerge, a 'reframing' in the sense that Deleuze and Guattari suggest, where the frame is open to what is beyond: "The painter's action never stays within the frame; it leaves the frame and does not begin with it" (Deleuze and Guattari, *What is Philosophy*, 1994, 188). For example, Iain MacRury tells the story of burly stand-up performer who takes the jibes cast at him in the outside world about his size and builds a comedy set around them, holding up those comments, and those who make them, for the audience's laughter (MacRury, "Humour as Social Dreaming", 2012; though see Chapter 14 of this book, concerning Hannah Gadsby and shame). The ritual of 'definitional ceremony' in narrative therapy seeks to acknowledge and reframe the client's life (White, *Maps*, 2007). Tony E. Adams writes about his father in order find different stories to tell about their troubled relationship (Adams, "Seeking Father", 2006). In the chapters of Part 3, I write into three familiar, perhaps taken-for-granted territories (ethics, reflection and the body) and find myself in each caught by writing's power to 'reframe'.

Chapter 9

ONCE UPON A TIME, A STORY HIT BACK[236]

Edinburgh, Spring 2015 and February 2018

This chapter is about the telling of personal stories in writing-as-inquiry and stand-up. It is a chapter about ethics. Are personal stories, including those about therapy, worth the trouble they cause? The personal stories I write return to confront me with the consequences of the choice to give them air. I argue back to them: how could I have kept you quiet? How could I not have told you? What else do I have but the capacity—no, the responsibility—to tell you? Oh, how noble, they answer; and how very, very convenient. Yes, well, you can be sarcastic if you want, I retort, but I have to take the risk to allow you stories to do the work that's needed. I can't afford not to; there's too much at stake. The argument continues; and I am tired of it. This chapter will see if I can take it somewhere generative rather than circular, as I examine whether the conceptual and ethical work that stories lay claim to are ever worth the cost.

I liked this title when I first found it in preparation for a conference presentation, and thought the abstract—largely as written above—meaningful and heartfelt. I could picture the scene I painted; I felt part of it. I was up for an argument with myself, up for the fight. My sense of circularity and stasis in relation to this issue was profound, like grid-locked traffic on the London orbital motorway—M25 syndrome, perhaps—and I was desperate to find a way out of it, to negotiate my way through, to push hard into the gaps and off the slip roads to find a no-doubt idealized highway where I could wind down the window and accelerate, carefree but purposeful, Bruce Springsteen turned up to the max. I was prepared to battle for it, to find a dominant position from which I could justify myself and continue to write the kinds of stories that I was calling myself out for.

Now that I have begun to write, I realize that neither the title nor the abstract serves me well. I still like them in their catchiness and energy, as far as that takes me, but they constrain me; and, I will argue, they constrain us. I say more about this later, but the key point is that both title and abstract risk buying into a notion of ethics as codifiable and governable, and into the binary of stories being either ethical or not; both ethics and stories as one thing or the other. As if stories, like my writing here now are not already and always entanglements of ontology, epistemology and ethics: ethico-onto-epistemological.[237]

* * *

As described in Chapter 3, in their respective stand-up sets Reginald D. Hunter tells the story of an intimate conversation with his elderly father, Holly Walsh reports on the sexual advice her mother gave her as a teenager, Katherine Ryan lets the audience in on the recent messy break-up of her relationship, and Lucy Beaumont spins stories of her friend, Jackie, who's in search of a husband.

I saw three of these performers in Edinburgh in 2014, and the fourth (Hunter) in southern England some years before. Re-visiting and witnessing these performances now, I look over my shoulder to see if the 'other' they talk about is here. They are. I can see them, see their faces, get a sense of their bodies, their size, their age, their material presence: Hunter's father, Walsh's mother, Ryan's ex-partner, Beaumont's friend.

In early 2018, as I write my way towards completing this book, Haroon Siddique's *Guardian* article reports on how British comedian Louise Reay is being sued by her former partner for apparently defaming him and breaching his privacy in her 2017 comedy performance, *Hard Mode*,[238] in which she refers to their relationship.[239] Siddique writes that Reay's fellow performers are speaking up for their warrant to draw from personal material, claiming the issue as important in upholding the right to free speech, and are taking action in support of Reay. Sofie Hagen, whose current show, *Dead Baby Frog*, concerns her abusive grandfather, says:

> I came to the conclusion that this is my life and my experiences and he has made his bed. Or rather, he has made my bed and now I have to lie in it, so

at the very least, I should get to talk about it. It is absolutely laughable how so many men loudly cry for freedom of speech when it regards their own desire to spew sexist, racist and homophobic opinions on stage in the name of 'satire' but as soon as a female comedian talks about her own experiences with men, it's suddenly 'wow, wow, wow, what about my reputation'.[240]

Hunter's father, Walsh's mother, Ryan's ex-partner, Beaumont's friend. I hear them shout, as a heckler might: "How could you? That was between ourselves. A private conversation. How could you do this?" But none of these conversations is 'private', Hagen might argue. There's always a politics.

At her performance, I imagine Ryan's former partner stands up, walks along the row and up the cheaply-carpeted stairs before turning to shout back, "How dare you wash our dirty linen in public? How could you do that?" In other words, "What gives you the right? What warrant do you have?" In my imagination, I turn back to the stage to watch the performers respond. They remain unruffled. They don't shuffle their feet, they don't hesitate, and they don't look away. They each find a response, along the lines: "Well, you have a point. But take it from the rest of us here that just laughed, that story I just told of us? It was funny". Except they would make it sharper than that. The subtext of this, or maybe the response they might give when not under pressure, might be: "Maybe our conversations were private at the time; and I can see that you're not happy that I'm telling everyone here. But, yes, were they funny? They were, weren't they? So the real question is: how did the stories I told of us *work*? What work did they do? Did they carry meaning? Where did the audience go with them? Was telling the stories worth the cost?"

I hear this response and am not convinced. The audience may be left wondering how much these performers care. How much do the 'others' of their stories matter to them? How mindful of consequences are they? Stand-up and research may, arguably, be bound by different ethical expectations, but similar questions pertain.

In his wonderful book on the use of narratives and fiction in research, Peter Clough tells a series of sharp, sad, engaging stories about northern English state school life.[241] The stories are based upon and draw from Clough's ethnographic research in such schools. One story, *Lolly*, responds to the multiple questions and challenges Clough received when he read and published the earlier stories, questions about warrant,

137

ethics and consequences. 'Lolly', a young man in his twenties, knocks on Clough's door at home to threaten him over the story that Clough wrote about his younger brother, *Molly*. Molly has since died in a bike accident, for which Lolly holds Clough ultimately responsible. Lolly's story is powerful, plausible, truthful, full of hovering revenge and implicit menace. It's a story of chickens coming home to roost.[242] A story about a story taking a hit.

Another story about a story taking a hit:

It's May 2014 after a session at the International Congress of Qualitative Inquiry in Illinois, USA, in a top floor room of the main conference building, the Illini Union. The panel I have co-chaired has explored collaborative writing as a method of inquiry, where I and my long-time writing partner, friend and collaborator, Ken Gale, have read our latest paper. The paper and the panel have both gone well; there's been a good crowd of appreciative colleagues. And now people are leaving. I exchange hugs and thank-yous with fellow panelists and gather my papers into my bag. I walk between two now-ragged rows of seats towards the far door.

A man I struggle to recognize approaches. He's familiar but I'm not sure from where. He asks if we can talk. He tells me that he has followed our work, Ken's and mine, over the years. He's read all of our papers. I feel good. He goes on:

"But I did want to talk to you about one. I read an early paper you wrote together, and there's your story of one of your counselling clients—Janice?"

"Yes, Janice, I think so . . ." I begin to feel less good.

"It disturbed me. I've read other papers you've done since and they've been fine. But that one, I was really upset. . . . I'm sorry to put you on the spot. But Janice, was she real?"

He stops for a moment and I prepare to respond. I don't know what I'm going to say. But before I can say anything he adds, "If she were real, if she were one of your actual clients, that bothers me. I've hoped not, because if she were, I've felt. . . . I don't know . . . about contacting your professional body. They need to know".

I haven't seen this coming. I hesitate. I can sense the depth and seriousness of his concern. I don't know how to answer his question.

I must find something. I look for it; my breathing becomes shallow. I reply: "Was she real? Well, she was based upon a real person".

That's all there is. I feel my response sounding insufficient. Arch. I feel compromised. I feel like I've not done myself justice, nor Janice, nor the colleague in front of me. But it's all I can muster.

He says, "Ok. Because if she were real, that would be . . .", and his voice trails off. "Next time, could you put in a note to tell the reader?"

A note to re-assure, I take it. "No clients have been harmed in the writing of this paper".

I have been thinking about this conversation since, wondering what to make of it, wondering where it may take us. I am writing this chapter in part because of this conversation. My colleague may read it. But is *he* real? Was he real? Have I fictionalized him? Fictionalized us? Is it good that I have? Have I fictionalized us sufficiently? Have I told the truth about our encounter here, in this text? Have I done him justice? Have I done us justice? What is 'real', anyway? Like the question I impute to comics Hunter, Walsh, Ryan and Beaumont, I must ask, what work does this story do? Is it worth the risk? Does the story demand being told?

If there were a problem in the original telling of the story of Janice, my client, all those years back, I am going to risk compounding it now. I am going to tell the story of the story of writing about her.

The story is one I write to Ken concerning my final session of six with Janice. She had come to see me about the troubled and troubling relationship with her daughter-in-law. I write about sitting in my consulting room soon after she has left at the end of the final session of our work together and I am despondent. I feel I have let her down, not been able to respond to her, not been able to 'help'. Janice is early sixties, white, depressed. I give you these descriptors now but wonder what they do. They tell you something; they give us the faint lines of an image we can create to still our curiosity. A shape to build her around, drawing from ourselves and our stories of the 'Janices' in our histories. In common ways of considering ethics, I am inviting you, as I did back then, to 'believe' me, to 'trust' that I am being 'honest', whilst also that I am honouring the contract I have with my client. Honouring her, honouring you, honouring me. Though I recognize that, for my colleague at the conference, this trust in me was not possible to find.

In the paper, I am telling the story of my work with her, this story of my despondency, to Ken. I write to him that I need to tell him, in order to work at the stigma, the wound, and to move on from it. To make sense of it, to not let it 'nail' me; or maybe to let it do so but not allow it to lead to a kind of death.[243] By writing it and, specifically, by writing it to/ for you I am looking for the 'promise of the text'[244] in its broadening of the struggle;[245] offering you the text as a searching for space where something different might occur.[246] The giving of it to you, when I click 'send' on the email, I am looking forward to that; not because I will find rescue but because this writing will lead us somewhere.

Somewhere we do not yet know.

Somewhere incalculable.[247, 248]

That is my justification. I am asserting that there is a wound that needs tending, that writing might do this, that writing *to Ken* might do this, and that there is the promise of relief—and the promise of purpose—in bringing this story to him and into our collaborative inquiry. Attention to the particular holds the hope that I, he, we, we all, might find change; something different might occur. That's my claim. That's why I say that it's worth telling Janice's story.

The story, one could say, hits back. Resists.

There are other stories. I see them returning to haunt me here.[249]

There, in the doorway—look. They enter, pause, stare; they fill up the rows of seats here, there, over there; they spill out across the room, some—real, not real, real enough—standing, arms folded, sceptical and angry; or wry, touched, amused, surprised, delighted. Both. All.

There—my brother and our sometimes-difficult relationship, about which I have written in the context of my loss of religious faith.

There—my father, whose stories I've written only since he died. Stories that don't only portray him at his best.

There—my daughter who, in her early teens, googled herself and found words she had thrown at me when she was ten quoted back to her in a story I tell. She never knew; I never asked if writing and publishing that story would be okay for her.

There—our son and his teenage gothic ways. At least I consulted him at the time.

There—my wife, often referred to, part of many other stories I tell and, sometimes, integral, as I work through and with the stories of our own relationship.

There—my mother, my sister, my friends.

They are all here too, in this book: father, mother, brother, sister, daughter, son, wife, friends. Some are mentioned only in passing; some (father, mother) dwell longer.

There—the man who drove me to Nairobi airport. I will give him his name again here. Rizile. Gift of god.

There—Terry, a counselling client, mourning his father. Petra: the client whose story prompted five of us into writing life together. Grant, too, and Amy, Tanya, Rosa. And—there—here, in this book—Karl. Rafa, too, later, in Chapter 12. Disguised, anonymized, consulted, 'fictional', or otherwise, these clients have life, they have body, in the text. They come to matter.

There are more stories of more others. What are the ethics of my not naming or not remembering them?[250]

All these have become 'characters' in or of my stories. I imagine them heckling me now, like those in the stand-up performers' stories. Some might claim I have wrested their narrative material and potential from their hearts and moulded them to my ends, enabling me to publish and extend my CV. "How do you square this? That conversation, that relationship, was ours; it was between ourselves. A private conversation, a private relationship. What suggests it is acceptable to tell others about it? What right do you have?"

And I ask myself, was it worth it? Was it? The stories ask, were we worth it?

Maybe those I have written about are indifferent. Maybe they feel flattered or recognized or amused. There are those who might not heckle; they might respond with a glance, or a smile, or a nod or they might, I don't know, just say 'yes'.

***

The metaphor of stories 'hitting back', in justification, against imaginary rebuttals does not work for me now. I challenge my title, which suggests a retaliatory dynamic, a violence that does not serve this matter well. Does not do those stories justice, nor me.

I must find a way out of this oppositional, constricting bind, but not in the way I thought I might when I wrote the title and abstract, the latter implying too simplistic a notion of the personal, too crude a concept of the humanist other and its separate, 'real' self/selves. The colleague who confronted me at the conference demanded to know whether Janice was 'real', which, if so, would make my publishing her story an ethical breach. I speculated, in turn, in writing here, whether the character of this colleague I had constructed was 'real'. But these questions of the 'real' (albeit ironically posed) suggest a conceptualizing of 'real' as concerning discrete, "molar identity",[251] but the 'real' for Deleuze and Guattari is "becoming itself, the block of becoming, not the supposedly fixed terms through which that which becomes passes".[252] Such a notion demands we think not in terms of whether he or she, or you and I, are 'real', but instead attend to, notice, what we can touch, as they pass, of the pulses and flows of becoming's speeds and affects.[253] What do we sense in these encounters? That's where 'real' lies.

Further, my title and abstract slip into too simple a binary between 'right' and 'wrong', into Badiou's institutionalized *contemporary* ethics;[254] too neat a slide into Deleuze's *morality*, the "system of judgment"[255] that we so often think of as ethics but which Deleuze contrasts with an ethics that is not either/or, not good/bad, not ethical or not, but "about the powers we have singly and collectively, to endure and engage in creative evolution".[256] This is an ethics that attends to our "material continuity and ontological co-implication with others, including non-human others".[257]

In such a view, the point is that we stand *within* what we do and what we are, and what is, becoming. Or, rather, we are *of* these. We are within our narratives, standing together with them, *of* them; with and of the others, material, human and more-than-human, we write about; co-implicated, entangled,[258] however those others are realized in the stories that we put our names to.

Deleuze writes, "Either ethics makes no sense at all, or this is what it means and has nothing else to say: not to be unworthy of what happens to us".[259] I often think of and with this assertion, puzzling over it, wondering if it is a counsel of passivity and an abnegation of responsibility. Today, finishing this chapter, a weight of other tasks lining up the other side of it and my mother waiting for me to visit, I see it as neither of these. Instead, I understand Deleuze as calling for stories not to "hit back" but as asking to be seen, witnessed, in all their fullness, complexity and nuance.

Deleuze, Badiou and Barad encourage me to stand—or sit, writing—here and not seek to put down the hecklers, who, after all, are both me and not-me, both here and not here. Instead, Deleuze and these others would suggest, "Stand, re-cast yourself and these others as co-implicated and entangled, and take account of the decisions, the 'cuts', you make in bringing them to the page. That's all; that's everything".

Comics Hunter, Walsh, Ryan and Beaumont, and I, can only stand here, together with our 'others', our participants, our audiences, our witnesses and readers, and ask ourselves Deleuze's question: "am I, was I, will I become, not unworthy of what happens to me? And how can I make it so?", before however it is that we respond.

NOTES

236 This chapter was first presented as a paper at the 2015 International Congress of Qualitative Inquiry, as part of a 'Spotlight' session curated by Bronwyn Davies, "Story-telling onto-epistemological and ethical practice".

237 Barad, *Meeting the Universe Halfway*, 2007.

238 www.louisereay.com/comedy

239 Siddique, "Comedians Say Case of Sued Performer", 2018.

240 Siddique.

241 Clough, *Narratives and Fictions*, 2002.

242 Clough, x.

243 Cixous, *Stigmata*, 2005.

244 Cixous, xiv.

245 Coles, *The Call of Stories*, 1989.

246 St. Pierre, "Deleuzian Concepts for Education", 2004.

247 Cixous, *Stigmata*, 2005, xii.

248 Gale and Wyatt, "Writing the Incalculable", 2007, 792.

249 They are 'haunting' in the sense of calling to account. Saltmarsh writes, drawing upon Derrida in reviewing Avery Gordon's book (*Haunting*, 2008): "[T]he concept of haunting has considerable analytic force. In one sense, it signifies a speaking back of past to present and future, in ways that cannot necessarily be contained or fully reckoned with". Saltmarsh, "Haunting Concepts", 2009, 540. These stories are not 'returning'; they have always been there, speaking back.

250 And what are the ethics, I ask myself, of my not providing citations to the publications containing those I have named? An appropriate reluctance not to compound further any arguable ethical breaches? A desire to not be brazenly self-referential? And/or a trace of shame, perhaps?

251 Cull, "Introduction", 2009, 7.

252 Deleuze and Guattari, *A Thousand Plateaus*, 2004, 262.
253 Cull, "Introduction", 2009.
254 Badiou, *Ethics*, 2002.
255 Deleuze, "Cours Vincenne", 1980.
256 Davies and Wyatt, "Ethics", 106.
257 Davies and Wyatt, 107.
258 See Barad, *Meeting the Universe Halfway*, 2007.
259 Deleuze, *The Logic of Sense*, 1990, 148-9.

Chapter 10

SHADOW BANDS

Thinking Therapy Diffractively[260]

Edinburgh, Spring 2015

How might Donna Haraway's notion of 'diffraction', and Karen Barad's develop-ment of this way of "rethinking the geometry and optics of relationality", affect what takes place in, and how we understand, the therapeutic encounter? And how might working with this concept impact upon how we view the established practices of clinical supervision, where the therapist and supervisor are tasked to 'reflect' upon the therapeutic encounter? In this chapter I will draw from the material of my own therapeutic and supervisory practice in exploring what happens when we begin to reframe the habitual.

13 MARCH 2015 ECLIPSE MINUS ONE WEEK

On this keen Scottish late-winter Friday morning—we have shifted our sessions to Fridays and to a different room for a couple of weeks to accommodate his travel commitments—I envy Karl and his thick leather coat. He reaches down to the dull, blue, abraded carpet and picks the coat up, heavy in his hand. He shuffles into it as he stands to leave.

"We'll see how it goes", he says. "I don't know if she'll be there when I get home. I hope she is. And I hope she isn't".

He turns and says thank you, I'll see you next week. "Or won't", he adds.

I don't understand and show that I don't. "During the total eclipse", he explains. He can see I'm doubtful. "The eclipse, when I'm here, after we start. About 9.30".

I'm surprised. I've forgotten. Or never knew. I haven't looked that far ahead.

"Ah yes", I lie. "See you then". He smiles, knowing, turns the handle on the door and leaves. And only when he's gone do I get the joke about not seeing me. It'll go dark, Jonathan, dark.

***

I still talk about reflection. With students, with fellow counselling practitioners, with academic colleagues. We just do, apparently. To say 'diffraction' feels an artifice, a pose, a clever play inviting the question "What do you mean, 'diffraction'?" whereupon I can give the concept a convoluted explanation (convoluted because I don't feel as if I inhabit it, can't shuffle into it, like a coat, with familiar ease); and if I'm lucky I sound well-read and intellectual.

Case in point: during the recruitment process for my current position at Edinburgh, when I presented on my research to a group of potential colleagues and students, I dropped in 'diffraction' with studied nonchalance. A member of the audience duly asked me to explain, and I duly responded with due inadequacy. As I could and should have predicted.

'Reflection' is a shibboleth in counselling and psychotherapy: it is woven through therapeutic discourse, as it is into all conversations about professional and pedagogic 'development'; it's seen as vital to good practice; it's the staple motherhood and apple pie diet of our 'growth' as practitioners. To talk in terms of diffraction sounds pretentious.

But I sense an urgency I don't yet understand. That we must; and we must do so now. Maybe I shouldn't worry and it's not that interesting; maybe it's only semantics: of course we mean the complexity that 'diffraction' implies, and not the metaphoric straightforwardness, the sameness, that reflection suggests. But that's not good enough: we know what discourse does, how it disciplines our thought, how it and we are entangled within material-discursive practices, how discourse *matters*. In this chapter, therefore, through telling vignettes of work with a client before and around the total eclipse in March 2015, and through theory, and through writing, and through stand-up—as these diffract, one through the other through the other—I want to see where diffraction might take me, take us, take the therapeutic and supervisory encounter; I want to see where diffraction might take us differently.

20 MARCH 2015 ECLIPSE MORNING

He's late, by twenty minutes. That's nearly half our time. The eclipse has been and all but gone. I stood by the window as I waited for him, feeling the morning turn cold, a dullness tinged with danger.

When I collect him from the lobby he's still in the black leather coat, breathing heavy, his forehead damp in the overhead light.

In our seats opposite each other, he places his hands on the armrests, looks down at his tie, and lifts a hand to smooth out a ruffle, which re-appears.

"Sorry I'm late. It was the eclipse".

"You waited to see it?"

"No. You don't do that, do you? You shouldn't. You don't 'see' an eclipse. You don't look at one, not without damaging your eyes". He articulates these words with precision, keeping his eyes down and his hands on the armrests. Like I'm not there, and, if I am, like I'm not that smart; and like I'm definitely not a scientist. I can't tell if he's being ironic.

"No, it wasn't me, it wasn't that", he continues. "The kids wanted to stay home for it before going into school, so they were dragging their heels. I half-heard on the radio—I was in the shower—that the eclipse would do that. Cause cars to break down, PC systems to fail, wars to begin. Slow down the metabolisms of teenagers. Make half the kids in the country late for school. No need to wait for the zombie apocalypse".

He doesn't smile but I laugh, then so does he.

***

Reflection casts an image back upon itself. In the bathroom in the morning, the Jonathan I look at in the mirror enables me to see myself 'as I am', baggy eyes, crags, lines, hair loss, new beard growth, filled teeth and all; when I clean my teeth and brush my hair my 'reflection' provides me with visual data that shows me 'what I am doing'. The mirror is neutral, I might believe, giving me back only what I give it; the mirror changes nothing, I say. The mirror doesn't lie; it can't. Mirrors don't lie. (Ask the queen in Snow White.) Like the witnesses to Wallace Stevens' *Man with the Blue Guitar* who demand that he play "things exactly as they are"—green— we see reflection as innocent, devoid of power, shorn of any impact that the ontological, epistemological and ethical practices in which we are engaged may have.[261]

Diffraction draws our attention instead to difference and effect. It isn't just that reflection is inadequate; and it isn't just that it's not what we mean. Reflection is a mirage, in this sense; it already changes. The image in the mirror is not me. It is partial and limited; it's reversed. It changes as I shift from one foot to the other; it's governed by the position of the bathroom light, affected by whether or not I am wearing my glasses; it's dependent upon what else I am thinking about as I gaze, how late I am, how steady my breathing is, how clean the mirror, how magnified, how positioned, how full I still am from last night's dinner or last night's argument, how anxious I am about the morning's trying meeting, how good about myself I feel, how much of my father I see in my face today and how much steam from the shower remains swirling in the haze around me. In the bathroom mirror I can never see myself from behind or above or the side. I can perhaps claim that I gain a glimpse of what my face offers to the world that morning; but not even that, only what it offers to me, then, in that instant.

Mirror, mirror, on the wall, who is the fairest of them all? "As if I know", replies the mirror. "As if 'knowing' is that kind of practice, held by one (me) and not another (you) and acquired through the visual. However, if you push me to answer your question", continues the mirror, "it's not you".

And as if there's a 'me' that can ask the mirror. As if there's a me that's inseparable from the mirror, from the image, from the space I'm in, from the space I am, from the time, the moment, the 'this-ness', the *haecceity*.[262] As St. Pierre might claim: "Representational schemas assume depth and hierarchy—first, that there is a primary, originary reality out there to be found and, second, that [reflection] can accurately represent it".[263]

So we must talk about and work with diffraction. We must. I must.

Because:

I see my client, he of the coat and the eclipse, on these Friday mornings. Ten minutes before he's due I look at the notes from the week before; they are highlights, perhaps, my brief summary of what seemed most important; my 'reflections'. The notes take me back and bring me forward. Sometimes, as I read those few lines, what I have forgotten returns to me: the way he talks, the gestures he makes, his early-morning, office-ready scent. I become re-acquainted with my sense of the other; and notice the turn my body makes in response, to hopeful, fearful, intrigued.

If I have time during those waiting minutes in the counsellors' office, and if the sun is out, I stand and look through the window into the garden, to its stone outer wall and, beyond, to the faint rise of the hills.

I talk with colleagues, perhaps, about the TV thriller we've been watching. I keep an eye on the clock on the far wall. When it's time, I open the door and turn right. I steer left around the corridor, smile at my client, who has sensed me arrive as he reads; he rises and I lead him to the room, holding open the door, then we sit and wait.

We must talk of diffraction because:

I go to supervision, once a month. All therapists have supervision. It is part of good, ethical, practice, enshrined in history and codes and principles and rules. We say we 'should', and that's no doubt right; but maybe it's another truism we might do well to hold open for diffractive attention. I 'take' my client to my supervisor. I tell her the stories he brings and I tell her of my responses. We hold all these between us: what my client said, what I said, what I felt, what I found myself thinking, what I feel now, what she, my supervisor, feels now. What gets called forth in and between us by the story of the client-and-me-in-the-room? Even this is inadequate, because by omission it implies that 'we', the 'humans', are all that matters as we sit and talk. It does not yet speak to the 'entanglements' that "reconfigure our beings, our psyches, our imaginations, our institutions, our societies";[264] those entanglements that 'we' are an inextricable part of and that become worked and re-worked in our therapeutic and supervisory encounters.

We must talk in terms of diffraction because 'reflection' is inadequate as a conceptualizing of all such events. So static. So dull. So binary. So linear. So limiting. So sluggish. It's not what we do and it's not what we mean.

***

Writing now, I am sluggish, distracted by everything. My cup of tea; my chocolate brownie; the sound of sirens; and by how, this Saturday afternoon in late March in our back room, I am watching the sun die on the angled wooden skeleton of a roof-in-progress. I want to look at the roof, not engage with diffraction and therapy. I want to look at how the scaffolding on the roof's near side glints; how the bare joists look like triangular chunks of a Toblerone; how I imagine a giant reaching down to scoop it up and crunch it in her eager mouth; how I would like to be that giant eating that giant honey-wooden roof-Toblerone, crunching my way through it as I bestride the Georgian tenements, lost in the moment of melting chocolate and tiny brittle nuts, before, through a ground-floor window nearby, I catch the enticing sight of a man on a sofa writing at his laptop, a laptop that looks like an after-dinner mint.

Maybe I, the man on his sofa writing at his after-dinner mint, am not distracted at all; maybe the giant and her appetite for confectionary, the whole surreal fantasy, is working at diffraction and therapy. "[B]elieving a thing's true/can bring about that truth", writes poet Alice Fulton, though I doubt she had Toblerones in mind.[265]

This morning I was reading Stewart Lee, where he declares that in his stand-up he wants there to be something at risk, something at stake; how he's always seeking to work at the edge of his capacity, daring himself to step into discomfort, into the threshold.[266]

Here, this, now, I have not yet nailed what's at stake; or I'm not yet aware that I have. I don't yet sense an edge within reach. I'm not working in the threshold; I (or the writing) will get there, I know, or maybe I am but I haven't yet clocked that I am, and for now I can only claim that I'm under a duvet on my sofa with tea, brownie and a giant. But I'll keep pushing, keep believing.

I'm seeing life, including therapy and including writing—especially therapy, especially writing—through stand-up, through Stewart Lee and his ilk. I can't help it. It's taken me over. Dazed and confused, I stumble through a world full of small, lit stages in darkened, mostly empty, rooms.

This preoccupation, this obsession, is troubling me but I think it helps too. Makes something possible, something new. As does taking in the view out of the window of the counsellors' office, as does telling stories to my supervisor, and noticing how the client picks up his coat, and the giant and her Toblerone. Stand-up—the stand-up-in-me, the stand-up-in-this—diffracts. It diffracts everything. It doesn't reflect. With diffraction, everything changes, everything breaks, disrupts, dismantles, becomes something different, something other.

Diffraction, writes Karen Barad recently, concerns "in/determinacy": "In/determinacy is an always already opening up-to-come. In/determinacy is the surprise, the interruption, by the stranger (within) re-turning unannounced".[267]

Like an eclipse, you can't look at diffraction, you can't see it, not directly. You let it take you over, imbue your world, suffuse your therapeutic practice, slow down your metabolism; you're better to open yourself to diffraction, together/apart, sensing the mystery, the interruption, the strange and the stranger, the giants and the zombies.

20 MARCH 2015, ECLIPSE MORNING, CONTINUED

"Do you know", he says, breaking the silence after our laughter, "that there are faint patterns of light and shadow, 'shadow bands', that can often be glimpsed for a few moments before and just after a total solar eclipse?"

"No, I didn't know that", I reply.

"Well, there you go. You heard it here first. No one knows what causes them, the shadow bands. Diffraction is one possibility".

"Diffraction".

"Yes. Maybe. Maybe not. It's a mystery".

I wait. We wait. The room waits.

"You seem different today", I say. "Or we do. I don't remember us laughing together. I don't remember either of us laughing".

"No", he says. "I don't laugh much. Not now. Here or out there. Did I say, she was there when I got home last week? I wasn't disappointed". Hesitates. A shift, a flicker, a faint movement between shadow and light. "Ah well, it must be the eclipse. Laughter is our shadow band. It appears then disappears and no one knows what it is or why".

"I like that. The shadow band".

"But we did laugh, didn't we?", he adds, reaching for something. "We laughed and, for those moments, it felt good".

NOTES

260 This chapter was first presented as a paper at the 2015 International Congress of Qualitative Inquiry, as part of a 'Spotlight' session curated by Bronwyn Davies, "From Reflexivity and Repetition to Diffraction and Differentiation".

261 Stevens, *Harmonium*, 2001.
262 Deleuze and Guattari, *A Thousand Plateaus*, 2004.
263 St. Pierre, "The Posts Continue", 2013, 649.
264 Barad, *Meeting the Universe Halfway*, 2007, 383.
265 Fulton, *Powers of Congress*, 2001.
266 Lee, *How I Escaped*, 2010.
267 Barad, "Diffracting Diffraction", 2014, 178.

CHAPTER 11

W/B/ROUGHT TO LIFE[268]

March–April 2016, Edinburgh

How does the notion of 'emergent intracorporeal multiplicity' disturb assumptions about the relational encounter? How does the counselling client I write about, Karl, emerge as I write and how does or does he not connect both with me and with the memories I have of other clients? How are his particularities—his voice, his turn of phrase, his dress sense, his work, his family, his life, the way in which we laugh together in the room—serving me and others? What work does he do (to use Ron Pelias's phrase)?[269] (And why does asking that question feel instrumental and disrespectful and reductive, when he is arguably fictional?) How do the aesthetics of how he is w/b/rought to life contribute to what we say: how do they matter? Can 'emergent intracorporeal multiplicity' help us think/feel our way into these conversations?

It wasn't always like this. Wasn't always so hard to see him. The shape of him, how he moves. Or hear him: the timbre of his voice, his edge of irony. Some days it has been like he's been there, in front of me. Right *there*. A stack of bones and muscle, ligaments and tissue: a cadence of breath and blood. All of him, like I could lean forward in my chair and—reach—touch; feel the warmth of a body. I never would, never could, bring myself to do so; but sometimes in the writing he has been like that. I want to say, sometimes he has been so *real*.

Today, though, I am losing him. He has faded. He shimmers, there, in that chair, beckoning, promising, but when I look for him he wanes, his shape fading into the off-white walls. I am no longer sure of him.

I am talking about Karl. Karl, the client I am writing about as I continue to work on how stand-up, therapy and writing speak to each other. Karl with the smart suits and the buttoned-up jacket and the sharp tongue. Karl, whose pain fills the room, there on the page and here as I write. Karl, whose family is crumbling and whose life is stalled. A middle-aged, professional man with young adult children. Karl who laughs and makes me laugh. White, British, middle-class, straight, 'able-bodied', sad, funny Karl. Karl, whose life I create, perhaps, in near enough my own image.

One take on Karl, through Kelly Fritsch, is that he is an example of an "ableist failure of imagination"; how, when I have been writing, it was *this* kind of a body that I created for Karl.[270] One that, apparently, functions in the realm of 'normal' and 'healthy', though who knows what is hidden that I am unable to see and who knows what he has not yet revealed. I do not craft him as having a body with disabilities. Disability, writes Fritsch, "remains a . . . profoundly undesirable category of being",[271] and I do not desire this for Karl just as I do not desire this for myself. I do not *not* desire this; I have not decided against it; I just do not think it. It does not fit my imagined narrative arc.

So, now, here he is. With me, but elusive. Like I no longer trust him, or trust myself. Maybe it is that as soon as we begin to know him as created, as made, as 'fiction', he loses his substance. As soon as our harsh gaze turns on him he shrinks back, not wanting to be found. "Of course", writes Peter Clough of the intimidating Lolly, "*Lolly* did not happen. But what is subtly terrifying about it is—to the extent that it 'works'—that it *could* have happened. Plausibility . . . is a key element here".[272] But it's not plausibility that's at issue here with Karl—I mean, he may be implausible, but that's not what is undermining my sense of him today. Karl *could* be happening, but it's worrying how he happens that is causing this.

Fritsch proposes that we see bodies not as individual properties but as 'emergent intracorporeal multiplicities', which, echoing Karen Barad's 'agential realism', "posits that bodies are formed *within a relation*, rather than formed 'across' or between already-formed bodies".[273] In these terms Karl is not only formed in relation to me and to his family, but I come to exist in relation to Karl. We make each other. Or, rather, our relating with each other—and, in Barad's terms, not our relating with each other as individuated human subjects but our entangled relating with and within the more-than-human and the material—leads to the emergence of our bodies.

> [B]odies are not simply in the world, but rather are engaged in a reconfiguration of what exists by intra-actively co-constituting the world. The dynamism of matter—human and non-human—brings forth new worlds.[274]

It is this broader claim of Fritsch's, of bodies being involved in "intra-actively co-constituting the world", that I wish to pursue here, to push at, to see if I can find a writing way into understanding, into *sensing*, her claim. Three stories follow in pursuit of this: of our son, my mother and Karl.

ONE

I am writing at my desk at home. I am alone in the flat. It is early morning on Thursday 3 March 2016. On Tuesday last week, 23 February, our son in Seoul was knocked off his bike by a truck.

It was his final week at work as a teacher of English, and his final week living in Seoul. He had been heading to the school via his usual route. In the account we heard first the incident occurred when he was cycling across a pedestrian crossing. This, we were told, is the norm in Korea. It wasn't that he was being irresponsible. He was wearing no bike helmet, also the norm. (Though how often did we admonish him as a boy, as he took off to school, for not wearing one? He would wear it until he was around the corner, then remove it and hang it on the handlebars. I know. I saw him one morning as I drove to work.) However, although he has no memory of the incident itself, and never will, he now says that he does not believe he had been on the bike. He would have been pushing his bike, walking beside it. He says this is what he always does.

This week he and his fiancée were due to leave Korea after four years to travel to Taiwan, Hong Kong, and elsewhere in the region, before heading to the USA in August to be married and settle. Now, ten days after the incident, he is out of ICU and in a general ward. Tess, his mum, left our home in Edinburgh on the day it happened and has been by his side since.

His brain bled. His brain is bruised below and behind his left ear, diagonally opposite where he experienced the impact when he fell, to the right and just above his right eye. He has not needed an operation. The scans reveal no lasting damage. Two days ago, his tubes were removed. He is recovering, restless and eager to be allowed to leave hospital. He is lucky. We are lucky.

Five thousand miles away I am maintaining daily routines of rising, working, eating, sleeping. I have been holding onto the familiar. I am walking between home and work, taking my usual route, twenty minutes up the steep hills in the mornings, fifteen minutes down in the evenings. But I take unusual care at Queen Street, where the commuter traffic is busiest, and at Princes Street, with its buses. While others make the decision to trust their judgement of relative vehicle speed, stepping into gaps, pausing in the middle as vehicles swing across them, I stand still on the pavement and await the summons of the green figure. In the long wait to cross I feel my imagination pull towards somewhere all that distance to the south and east, to what it would have been like for our boy and his body to have been one moment on (or beside) a bike traversing a familiar pedestrian crossing, thinking perhaps about the day's tasks and anxious about the endless infuriating bureaucracy of visa applications, aware of his longing to be away and somewhere other than this. Another breath, a half-breath, a step, a lift of toe and heel, a dip forward. The moment lost, superseded, becoming something other; a rupture, a shattering, a brutal encounter with concrete and metal, a grounding of dust and blood. Meanwhile, this body, mine and not mine, his and not his, waits for the eternally lithe green figure to flash before stepping off the pavement. Even as the signal summons me, I pause mid-crossing, when a movement to my left suggests a vehicle might be late in turning, its driver late for work and fretful. It's not. There is no car. My body is over-alert, over-attuned to unexpected movement. I no longer trust. Trust is a fantasy I have had to abandon, though it will have to return. To live without trust—however unfounded—is unsustainable.

Two

I arrive for lunch at the home on Mother's Day as arranged. At reception, it's Mickey I see first as he scurries towards me. As I crouch to ruffle his fur I see Mum across the lounge, edging her walker towards me. When she greets me she says, "You're going to be cross with me when I tell you this but until I just saw you I had forgotten you were coming". I reply, "How could you? I was only here yesterday?" Although I am smiling when I say this, I mean it; and I realize it's not tactful. I have travelled a long way to see her. My awareness of her failing memory does not prevent me from expecting her to remember. She seems not to notice my irritation and hears only my playfulness, but I feel ashamed. She hesitates, then reaches out to hold my arm and says, "It's such good news about Joe being on the mend. I have been so worried". She has been calling or texting every day since the accident. She has held on each morning to her awareness that the now grown-up small boy, who played at her house for hours with my childhood wooden toys, is laid out on a hospital bed, hurt. My short visit yesterday may not still be with her, but the self-contained grandson from all those years ago is.

She sends me to find a seat and order her pre-Sunday lunch drink while she "sees to something". I find a space and watch the residents gather, each of them, in painful slow motion. When Mum arrives she parks her walker alongside others lined up like a taxi rank and grasps my elbow as we weave between wheelchairs, sticks and tables to the chairs I have found. Mum grimaces as she grips the armrests before dropping into her seat, Mickey jumps onto her lap, she reaches for her sherry, and in that moment she seems almost happy. Almost. "Disability is a practice", writes Fritsch. "As an intracorporeal practice, disability is a life worth living".[275]

As I stretch out my legs, I imagine how it will feel for my body to lose ease, which if I live long enough it surely will.

THREE

Karl looks across at me, like he does. Eyes narrowed, like he has spotted something I haven't seen. He looks away, then back.

"There's something up", he says, finally. "You're not here. Not like usual".

"Say more. What do you mean?", I ask.

"You seem tired. Or distracted. Or something. Like you don't want to be here".

How can he tell? I thought I was doing a good job of putting all this to one side.

"I'm fine. Thanks, Karl. Where would you like to start?" An attempt to hold onto what I see as being the task. Him, not me.

"Yeah, right".

"What would it be like for you if I were those things, Karl? If I weren't tired or distracted?"

"It would be surprising. You'd be surprising. You'd be like the rest of us, a sentient, human being. Which I know would be a struggle for you".

It's dark outside, the white blinds only half-down so that in the ten minutes in between Karl and my next client I can open the window. The low lamp on the table is on, the tall lamp behind Karl is lit, and one more at the back of the room by the door behind me. A three-way glow of dim, quiet despair. I take a slow, deep breath and decide.

"My son is in hospital a long way from here, abroad. A truck collided with him on his bike. His mum is with him. She has been there since it happened. He is recovering".

Karl is still. I don't look at him. I go on.

"And I'm sad, and scared".

I look at him now. His face seems soft, somehow, like he's lost the edge he wears.

"Well, shit", he says. "No wonder you're not here".

"But I am. I am".

The two of us, him and me, and my boy, there; all of us in the half-light, broken.

NOTES

268 This chapter was first presented as a paper at the 2016 International Congress of Qualitative Inquiry, as part of a panel on "The Emergent Intracorporeal Subjects of Writing", curated by Bronwyn Davies.

269 Pelias, "Performative Writing Workshop", 2007.

270 Fritsch, "Desiring Disability Differently", 2015, 44.

271 Fritsch, 44.

272 Clough, *Narratives and Fictions*, 2002, 381.

273 Fritsch, "Desiring Disability Differently", 2015, 52, emphasis in the original.

274 Fritsch, 54–5.

275 Fritsch, 65.

INTERVAL

Towards Creative-Relational Inquiry (3): The Poetics of the Hyphen

In the first Interval I referred to creative-relational inquiry's "hyphenated" encounters. I ended the second interval by making a claim in creative-relational inquiry for a hyphenated personal, a hyphenated 'you'. In this brief third interval— an interval both in and out of time[276] and replete with sound: a note-in-itself[277]—I consider further the work the hyphen does within and for the concept of creative-relational inquiry. This writing is poetic, interrupted. I bring the hyphen explicitly into play again in Chapter 12, writing about shame.

Creative-relational inquiry is inquiry that puts its hyphen to work:[278]

> The hyphen as connection and link
> The hyphen as vibrant, as catalytic, as engaged
> A line, not a point
> a hyphen-line that is "bifurcating, divergent and muddled"[279]
> indicating
> not singular direction
> but unfolding
>   unpredictable
>   possibility
>
> A line that ties
> A line that joins
> A line that opens thinking into a "coming-into-relation of difference"[280]
> A line that speaks of engagement

The hyphen of creative-relational inquiry speaks of intimacy:

> A troubled, troubling, intimacy
> It pulls together and pushes apart
> The hyphen is not comfortable or comforting
> The hyphen is not cosy
> It plays with distance and proximity
> is suggestive of intimacy and hints at unease
> I might see the hyphen where you don't

Like:

Hyphens

> You talk together-talk
> like lace-tie teeth-clean
> no-thought pie-easy trip-off-the tongue
> and groove-like-Travolta

> You talk together-talk
> like mean-it believe-it
> heart-bottom on-mother's-life
> and so-help-me-god

> You talk together-talk
> like this is never-before
> lifetime-million-to-one-special
> and so-glad-I-found-you

> You do together
> like didn't see you there
> you get in my way crowd me
> and need space or never coming back

> Or is it I see together
> like hip-joined peas-in-the-pod
> sofa-curl dinner-for-two
> and hear hyphens you never use

The hyphen as push and pull, as tension, as force:

The hyphen speaks of power
it calls inquiry to be mindful of its own power
mindful of the processes of power within and beyond it
alert to how these shape and are shaped by inquiry
shape and are shaped by the bodies involved

The hyphen drives the creative-relational:

The hyphen is desire[281]
that's where its energy lies
never allowing inquiry to be complacent
always encouraging it to consider what's at stake
where it is
what work it's doing
what it's missing
what it's assuming and where else it might go

The hyphen does not privilege one over the other
the creative over the relational
nor the relational over the creative
but privileges the possibilities they offer in their constant movement
their uncertainty
their working together.[282]

The hyphen of creative-relational inquiry keeps inquiry ready
alert
it opens
—stretches—
inquiry
to the limits

Notes

276 Noting how 'time' is not sequential but enfolded in/as past-present-future.
277 Noting how the interval between two musical notes is not a 'gap', empty, but has its own effect/affect.

278 Fine, "Working the Hyphen", 1994.

279 Deleuze and Parnet, *Dialogues II*, 2002, viii.

280 Manning, *The Minor Gesture*, 2016, 11. Manning here is discussing the hyphen of 'research-creation'.

281 See p.42, first Interval: "Desire is the push and pull, the draw, the force of the creative-relational; the force that connects, the force that leans us towards (the) other, towards becoming-other, towards movement, towards change".

282 However, I note how Lisa Mazzei and Alecia Jackson discuss their preference for the double arrow over the hyphen in their use of Karen Barad's key term, 'material<-->discursive', as a move to avoid giving one 'half' more weight than the other. Mazzei, "Beyond an Easy Sense", 2014; Mazzei and Jackson, *Thinking with Theory*, 2012.

Part 4

Reframings (Continued)

Shame[283]

---

283 This final part of the book continues the 'reframing', in Deleuze and Guattari's sense, of Part 3. The three linked chapters in Part 4 dwell—uneasily—with shame. In writing these chapters, I have found Jackson's conceptualizing of "thinking without method" as happening through encounter, by force, and by chance, to be crucial in the writing-work of reframing, in particular in the thinking that was enabled in writing's encounter with the Cailleach (Jackson, "Thinking Without Method", 2017).

CHAPTER 12

TWO STORIES OF SHAME

Calling Upon the Cailleach

Spring 2017, Kilcreggan

This is the first of three chapters in which I diffract three stories of shame. In this chapter, I tell two of these stories: I offer first the story of performing a stand-up set in 2016 in which I tell the audience about a client, Rafa, and the impact of that performance. I move on to speak about another stand-up evening, when my own performance was not a success. Neither Rafa nor I come out of these respective stories well. The first story prompts me to consider how I might have been shaming of, perhaps cruel towards, Rafa. The second—my stand-up disaster—takes me into an encounter with my own shame. In the chapter I draw from Elspeth Probyn's writing about (writing about) shame; and I call for assistance on the Cailleach, the Celtic storm goddess. A third, connected, story of shame follows in Chapter 14.

A First Story of Shame

It's June 2016. I'm in Dundee, sitting on a bar stool with my eyes closed. I'm here to perform my second eight-minute set for the first time. An hour to go and the bar's basement performance space is still empty. The night's five other performers are here too, sitting at this end of the room by the improvised stage, a wooden block brought in for the night. Behind it, and to my left, is a drape with 'Bright Club' in red and yellow, and an image of the Bright Club duck.[284]

My fellow performers are talking, as was I till just a moment ago. Now, I need to retreat, and I sit back on the stool against the wall and close my eyes. Earlier, I'd walked from here up the hill and around and between various university departments, including a Maths block, an Engineering building and one where students were working in some state-of-art high-tech suite. It will have been a wealthy department, no doubt. Medical Sciences or the Business School. Whichever, I was envious. I walked and breathed, trying to get the breathing deep. I told myself it didn't matter how my set went; and that there wasn't much I could do to control that either. Somehow, these events seem to have a life of their own and not much of it is to do with what I do or don't do, or imagine I do or don't do.

So, now, I retreat, again noticing my breath. And wait. Over the next while I variously sit forward and re-join the conversations, head out for another walk, visit the bathroom (twice), talk to the only two people I know when they arrive as the room fills, and attempt to stay in touch with my calm though I know I am terrified.

I am the third act. I follow a performer whose ethnographic research looks at the connections between culture, politics and major weather events. She calls herself 'Disaster Girl', throwing her hand in the air and striking a convincing superhero pose. Her final story concerns being out in an electrical storm and falling into a large cowpat on the walk back across fields. When she travels home on a train afterwards, she finds herself having to explain her look and 'scent' to offended fellow travellers. She recounts to us how she tells them, "You see, I'm Disaster Girl and I was just walking across a field".

The MC, Susan Morrison, does a neat link, somehow, between weather superheroes and therapy, calling the audience to cheer the next act onto the stage, announcing my name and the title of my set in the usual whooping and clapping that all but drowns out her voice each time. I slow myself onto the stage, detach the mic, lift the stand out of the way, and begin:

Stand-Up: Counselling on Legs[285]

Good evening. I'm Jonathan Wyatt. I'm a lecturer in counselling and psychotherapy at Edinburgh. Though maybe not for much longer.

It has its drawbacks, being a therapist. People expect too much of you. They expect you to have everything worked out, they expect you to be sorted.

They expect you to have your shit together. Like my client said to me the other day,

"But *you're* meant to have your shit together".

And her husband said to me that afternoon:

"You're the one who's meant to have your fucking shit together".

And the nice policeman said to me: "Dr Wyatt, just go home. And get your shit together. Er, no, no . . . no, you can't keep the handcuffs. No, not even for 'therapeutic' purposes".

But being a therapist has its benefits, too: I'm no good in the sack, but I can talk about it. I'm good at that. My wife says I'm being hard on myself. Which is kind of tactless. She says I'm better than I think. She says I'm not just *good* at talking about it, I'm excellent.

I'm a therapist and my research is about what happens in the consulting room. It's a complex process. There's always so much going on. As a way to think about this, what I'm writing about at the moment are the parallels between therapy and stand-up.

The first connection is you go to both to feel better. There are things going on in your life, things from your past you want to sort out. Maybe it has been difficult for a while, and you go to a therapist. You spend a while there—a few sessions, a few months, a few years—and when you finish you feel better.

Just the same in stand-up: there's some things going on in your life. Maybe you've had a hard week at work, you need to get out of the house, whatever, and you're feeling like you need to let off steam, get a different perspective. You go out, have a few drinks, chat to a few people, have a few laughs, and go home feeling better. And if it's gone really well the audience goes home feeling better too.

Another parallel: in both stand-up and therapy people talk about really intimate things. Reginald D. Hunter tells this story about driving in a car with his dad and asking his dad whether he's ever had anal sex. (Whether his *dad* has, that is. Not whether his dad knows whether he, Reg, has had anal sex. That would be weird, because it's the sort of thing you'd think Reg would know. And his dad not to know.) But consider that though: that Hunter actually *did* ask his dad that question; and now, with an audience, he's admitting he did.

It's the same in therapy. You find yourself with someone you trust and you know what you say won't go anywhere else, you know you won't be judged. You find yourself able to talk about things you've maybe never told anyone else before.

In both people say the unsayable. There are limits, though. I mean, I may admit to you that I'm not good in bed, but I'd never tell my therapist. However good I am at talking about it.

But what's driving my interest in this most is how both require being *in the moment*. In both you've got to be alert to what's happening in the room, the vibe, what's going on, what's needed; alert to finding just the right words at just the right time and say them in the right way. So right now, here, there's something at stake, and none of us quite knows what's going to happen. I might forget where I'm going with this. I might drop the mic. I might die. Or I might get it spot on with a line and laughter will take us over. (You may have to use your imagination.)

Well, it's the same in therapy. Like my client, Rafa, yesterday evening.

I've been seeing Rafa a few weeks, and I could tell from the way he walked in that he was down. He told me what had happened. On Friday afternoon, he went to the cashpoint but it wouldn't give him any money. ("Fuck off, Rafa".) So he went into the bank itself. They wouldn't give him any more cash either because he's too overdrawn, and he isn't being paid till next week. ("Fuck off, Rafa".)

He was so angry and humiliated, he didn't go back to the flat where his girlfriend was waiting. Instead he went down the road to the pub and sat at the bar and had a drink, and then another. Some friends came in and they got the story out of him and felt sorry for him. They did what good friends do and they bought him more drinks. There was a girl there he likes and they ended up having a kiss.

He got back to the flat much later than he'd said and his girlfriend was still there, sitting in the kitchen. He was drunk enough not to realize he shouldn't tell his partner what had happened, and especially about the kiss, so he did. Of course, she was furious and upset and hurt, and she reached out and picked up a vase on the side. It was the vase his mother gave him, that's been in the family for generations, a Joseon porcelain vase, no less, and she'd given it to him just a few months before she died a couple of years back.

(Look, I realize this isn't a very happy story. But I don't have clinical supervision for a few weeks so it's helpful to tell you. Thank you. Also, you're a lot cheaper.)

Rafa could see what was about to happen and he didn't say anything. He knew he deserved it. He turned as she threw the vase and it hit him on the back and dropped to the floor, splintering and scattering in pieces across the terracotta tiles; and he looked down and could see from the top of his eyes as she left the room and went into the bedroom. He heard a suitcase drop onto the bed and a few moments later she was at the kitchen door.

Meanwhile he was kneeling on the floor gathering together the broken pieces—very symbolic—and she gently threw her keys and they landed in amongst the fragments. Then she walked along the wooden hallway and he heard the door close quietly behind her. She didn't slam it.

Now he's here, in front of me, and he hasn't heard from her since, and his head is in his hands; occasionally he looks up at me as if to implore me to take this weight off him. I know I can't. I can feel the despair in the room, the loss, the grief, the anxiety, the shame, the self-hate; and I know that I need to say the right thing, find the words. I know I can't make it better, I know there's no silver lining, I know reassurance won't help. It's something else that's required: a presence, a way of indicating that I'm a witness to his distress.

There's silence. It's important to leave the silence, to not rush in, not to say something just for the sake of it. I think about how his mother left the family home when he was small—she came back soon after—and I wonder if there are any echoes of that in this experience. And I think about how I was away a few weeks back and he'd found that difficult—clients get attached to their therapists—and again I think about how this maybe has echoes. I wonder whether it might be helpful to make these connections. But it doesn't feel right. Such interpretations just feel glib.

So, I'm here, in the moment, this broken, regretful young man and me in a dull-lit room in a non-descript building in a quiet Edinburgh suburb on an early Tuesday evening, and I look to stand-up for help: I become alert to timing, to notions of truth, to vulnerability, and I say:

"Rafa, I can see that this has been an awful time for you. But—and I want you to look at me here: it's time you got your shit together".

I've been Jonathan Wyatt, counsellor. Thanks for listening.

***

That was June 2016. Jump forward to May 2017.

You have to start writing somewhere. I began this at home on dark mornings in March, unable to see more than the street-lit courtyard beyond the window. I finish it as the days have lengthened towards early summer in a living room in Kilcreaggan, in the west of Scotland, where light enters through windows on three sides. When we arrived three evenings ago after the two-hour drive west from Edinburgh, I could see through the window facing southwest, which stretches the width of the room, all the way across the Clyde estuary below the house to the mountains of the Isle of Arran in the far distance, the glowing sky arcing to meet them. This afternoon the air is heavy, and the clouds are dropped low over land and water, where they have lain each day since.

Sometimes, as you'll see, it's enough to make you long for Celtic storm goddesses and their fury to clear the air so you can hold your head up straight and breathe.

You have to start somewhere. 'Start', an indication of movement, of action. Writing as a start, less a marking from stasis to dynamism, less the ignition of a car, the moment of the engine beginning to turn, less a decision, after weeks of hesitation, to start writing. 'Start': more how the wind fills the sails as the tiller turns, lifting the prow and gathering speed.

***

As excuses go, "I am researching the connections between stand-up and therapy" is not the most convincing reason for venturing on stage. It requires commitment, though. If I had wanted to try my hand at stand-up, to find an outlet for the performer in me, I could have just given myself permission to do it. I did not need to start writing a book that has taken as long as this to write. I didn't need the cloak of a 'serious' reason to want to be on stage. "It's ok, Jonathan", I could have said to myself, "you're allowed to want to have a crack at it. Just go and do it". Putting my name down on the list for an open mic night would have been perhaps more honest and more direct. And it would have been over in five or ten minutes and would have involved less labour.

There are parallels here with therapy. I did not need to justify seeking my own therapy by tying myself into six years of training to be a therapist. When I told my therapist at our first session over twenty years ago, "I'm here because it's part of my training", he replied, "Well, let's see how this goes. After a while we might discover why you're really here". We did; it didn't take long.

Three years into writing this book and I am sure my future does not lie on the stage, especially after the recent venture in early December 2016, when my five minutes did not go well, more of which later in this chapter. I have not been back on stage since.

A little less than a year ago, I wrote and performed the eight-minute set above, "Stand-Up: Counselling on Legs" at Bright Club in Dundee. I performed it again later in 2016 in both Glasgow and Edinburgh. It is the second set I have written and performed. I performed the first set, in which I tell stories of my father and of mishaps as a therapist, four times in 2015 at comedy events in Scotland and northeast England.[286] In this second set, which I am going to revisit briefly now as a lead into thinking about shame, I wanted to try something else, to push further, to take greater risks.

The set begins with my bemoaning the assumptions people, including clients, often make that therapists, *because* they're therapists, have or should have their life sorted. People expect therapists, I say in the line that holds the set together, "to have their shit together". I give an example from my own clinical work: the client who challenges me with, "But I thought you were the one who was meant to have your shit together". The scenario ends with the tolerant police officer telling me to "just take your belongings, go home, and get your shit together, Dr Wyatt".

My complaint about these unreasonable expectations of therapists is, of course, one I both mean and do not mean. I am aware it is likely I am projecting and it is only me who feels I should have my shit together. Others know I don't, and know they don't, and they do not expect anything different from either of us.

The heart of the set then proposes ways in which therapy and stand-up are alike—they are both about making you feel better;[287] they both deal, at least sometimes, with the intimate; people say the unsayable in both;[288] and they both require being alert to the moment.[289]

To illustrate this final similarity I tell the story of working with a client in therapy, a young man I call Rafa. I say I've been working with him for some weeks and I saw him just yesterday. He was despondent because life took a terrible turn at the weekend. He realized he'd run out of cash on Friday, was refused any more by the bank, in response to which he'd gone to a bar to drown his sorrows with what he had left in his pocket.[290] While there, he kissed someone he shouldn't have, returning much later to the apartment he shares with his girlfriend and in his inebriated state revealed his indiscretion. Devastated, furious, she left and he hasn't heard from her since.

So, I say, bringing us back to yesterday's therapy session, Rafa was in the room with me and I was stuck. It was a crucial moment in the therapy session, with much at stake. I was with a despondent young man, who was full of shame and regret, and I did not know how to respond. I looked to stand-up for help, I say, because in stand-up you have to make judgements in the moment, in the thick of it, and that is what was required from me as a therapist in the here-and-now with Rafa. I turned for help to stand-up for its attention to truth and to vulnerability and for its capacity to find the right words and to say them in the right way at the right time. This helped me find how I needed to respond to Rafa, who was sitting with me, head in hands.

You know this, and you know the rest: "Rafa"—I am telling the audience this is what I said in the therapy room—"Rafa, I can see this has been an awful time for you. But—and I want you to look at me here[291]—it's time you got your shit together".

It gets a laugh. The laugh it gets is maybe not worth, or commensurate with, the lengthy, shaggy-dog build-up, but it nevertheless seems a satisfying way to end in its calling back to the beginning of the set. Anyhow, my eight minutes are up. I thank the audience and leave the stage.

The set was filmed and the evening's organizers posted it on YouTube. I sent the link to friends and colleagues. I asked for responses. One, Sarah, a good friend, and herself a therapist, emailed:

> Hmmm, not sure, to be honest. I think the opening minutes are really good, but the punch line at the end troubles me. I think if I were to look you up, because I'd like to go into therapy, and found you on YouTube, I might fear your riposte. There is something quite cruel about it; it seems to play into a fantasy of being judged, as client, and found lacking. I think we often hear clients' superego urging them to 'get their shit together', so to have that substantiated feeds paranoia. And yes, I know that the guy is a fabrication,

and that we can think all things imaginable about our clients, but to expose that beyond the therapy world is tricky. There is thinking it and acting it— this crosses a boundary, I fear, which made me feel quite uncomfortable.

I had not expected this response. It brought me to a halt. This is a story, her comments suggest, not only of Rafa's shame, which I had been aware of, but of an exploitation of that shame, which I had not been: a story of showing up, of ridicule. Her responses call into question the ethics of sending up therapy publicly in this way and the ethics of exposing this client, Rafa, who is (arguably) a fiction but yet who I and maybe others come to feel for. Implicitly, there is a challenge to how the milieu of stand-up allows for not the unsayable, but the cruel, to be spoken.

Whereas for the first performance of my first set I wanted all those around me—friends, colleagues, students, family—to come along, I performed this set for the first time in Dundee, a long way from home, and did not tell anyone in Edinburgh, including Sarah, I was doing so. I must, at some level, have sought that distance and anonymity. Maybe I was just being self-effacing, or did not want those who knew me see me bomb. Or maybe I knew it would be provocative.

Sarah's response left me thinking further about the dynamics and politics of humour: at whom or at what is the audience being invited to laugh? At Rafa? And/or at me? And/or at therapy? Laughing at ourselves as therapists and at therapy, and others doing so, and laughing at ourselves as clients or, even, at and with our clients, may well be a sign of our health and the health of the therapeutic work, an indication of our capacity to celebrate the creativity of our clients, ourselves and the therapeutic encounter.[292] However, where, when, how, who and who with?

Sarah's insight that we think and feel things as therapists we do not necessarily give voice to is accurate. I feel impatience, anger, boredom, irritation, delight, love, attraction and more. Of course, at times, I bite my tongue. And, of course, in the room, what I do when the capacity is there is not to speak directly of my impatience, say, but to hold such affective responses in mind, think about them, think *with* them, make use of them to understand what is being evoked in me that might tell me about my client, their world, and/or us, and help me find a way to offer something useful when the time comes.[293] Of course. And this is taxing work and tough to do and I do not always have the wherewithal to be able to do it and instead I sit there frustrated and trapped and silent, wanting to retreat from the intensity of the moment but doing my best to stay.

Or. This agonizing may be too much. At times—with thought and care (so, of course, not in public, not at a stand-up event)—directness in therapy might be what is needed. The constructive, if loaded, work of confronting might sometimes be called for. My therapist, more than once, all but told me it was time I got my shit together.

I will come back to Rafa.

A SECOND STORY OF SHAME

I turn now to a different stand-up performance. A five-minute stand-up performance of mine that did not go well. That lasted for more than five minutes. Which is in part why it did not go well.

This chapter moves across time and space. Here, it is still May 2017 and I am still in western Scotland, in that room with windows on three sides, writing under low clouds.

Last week I told the details of the story that follows for the first time. It has taken me five months to speak of it. It needed time, a glass of wine, the company of friends, and their kind, ironic, curiosity. The irony was present because, after all, we knew it was only stand-up. No one needed to take this too seriously. My friends didn't, nor did I.

It's only stand-up: hold onto that as you read, no matter what I tell you.

5 December 2016, at The Stand in Edinburgh. Comedy has a word for what happened, a word that's blunt, brutal, uncompromising and melodramatic: on 5 December 2016, I died.

It was a temporary death, of course, but not everyone resurrects. I have not been back on stage since, though I tell myself it is not because of what happened. No, I have been too busy, too scattered and too focused upon writing a book about therapy, stand-up and writing. It's not that I couldn't get back on stage. It's not that I wouldn't want to, at some point. No, I just haven't had the space. Yes, it's true I haven't been back to The Stand since, not even to see a show, let alone perform, but I could. If I wanted. It would be fine. It just, well, hasn't happened.

You hear how dying on stage happens to everyone, but there, then, on stage that evening in December 2016, the universality and ubiquity of on-stage death was no consolation. It felt unique and personal, much like mortality itself.

Berlant and Ngai, critiquing and problematizing comedy, write how not being found funny can pierce deep:

> If we have conflicting views of what should produce empathy, if we don't finally feel it for the same things, we can find each other shallow and prefer ourselves—but it's different to disrespect what gives someone pleasure as funny. It's experienced as shaming; as condescending; as diminishing. It may be that we hold our pleasures closer than our ethics. Or it may be that we understand that, mirror neurons aside, empathy's objects are the effects of training whereas comedic pleasure involves surprise and spontaneity and therefore we take its contestation more personally, as an interference with a core freedom.[294]

At The Stand, on stage in that familiar basement room, which I had previously found welcoming and forgiving, the faces and bodies contested my comedic pleasure in front of me, so close I could reach out and touch them, and drifted further and further away as I sank. Comedy loss circulates: fast, inexorable, ruthless.

***

Writing about shame, as Elspeth Probyn says, affects us in particular ways.[295] Writing this, now, with arms pulling away from the keyboard, eyes drawn to the window and a soon-to-be-summer-lush garden in Spring, 2017: "look", the garden calls, "look, listen, come feel the living here". A desire to do anything other than write. Doing the dishes, cleaning the toilet. There's a familiarity, of course, about the drawing away, the lure of somewhere different. It's not like I haven't referred to it elsewhere in the book; this reluctance is not unique to writing about shame. But there are particularities to this writing now. I notice a tension in my fingers as I press the keys that form the word 'shame', how I avoid saying the word to myself; how reluctant I am to begin putting any words onto the screen because then they will be *there*. How my breathing becomes shallow, my diaphragm rigid. Even when my shame was, on balance, inconsequential.

Writing earlier about Sarah's stark suggestion of my cruelty towards Rafa my fingers and belly eased. My arguable casting of another into shame felt easier to stay with; it felt easier to keep at this desk, fingers at the keys. To consider myself as, possibly, cruel is simpler to place aside. It is another, Rafa, I diminish and, well, I am reluctant to say, cruelty towards another does not strike so deep as my own shame. Probyn writes:

> If we want to invigorate our concepts, we need to follow through on what different affects do, at different levels. The point needs to be stressed: different affects make us feel, write, think, and act in different ways. Shame, for example, works over the body in certain ways. It does this experientially—the body feels very different in shame than in enjoyment—but it also reworks how we understand the body and its relation to other bodies or, for want of a better word, to the social. This matters at the level of theory. It matters in terms of what we want writing to do.[296]

Sometimes, I prefer not to understand my body and its relations to others, how the moving, multiple body is always and already implicated. But here I attempt to take up Probyn's call, to fold these stories into her invocation of what writing shame does.

The 5th of December, 2016, The Stand Comedy Club, Edinburgh. A Monday night. Red Raw—new material night. I love The Stand and I love what it stands for. A champion of new acts and, in particular, women performers from its inception, The Stand has always insisted, over twenty years, on there being at least one woman on the bill every night (rare twenty years ago), and it embraces edgy, radical, progressive comedy and its deep, dark, basement energy. The staff are warm, the vibe is safe. In general. It's still stand-up. It's still Red Raw.

The majority of the stand-up I have performed has been Bright Club, stand-up organized and performed by academics doing stand-up about their research to an audience mostly of others in the academy. (There was that surprising hen party at Bright Club one night.)[297] The Bright Club audience is kind and tolerant and ready to laugh at the comic possibilities of an obscure and untranslatable German term, the behaviour of a strain of bacteria or the connections between stand-up and therapy. Red Raw is a different beast, where comics, established or new or on the way, cut their performing and new material teeth. The audience is a general comedy audience, there for a good, cheap (£2) Monday night out. So, some students, yes, but even they, or especially they, are not there to hear about someone's latest research project. They are there for the comedy, whatever that means to them.

I first did Red Raw in July 2016. I was given five minutes, the usual limit you're given when you start, for which I adapted and compressed (so to speak) the 'shit together' material I had previously done for Bright Club. Frankie Boyle, arguably Scotland's favourite, certainly its most notorious, present-day comedian, was on the running order. He came and went via a side door, complete with minder. My five minutes ended up being only four—I didn't need to rush, it turned out—and I got a few laughs. It went fine.

The Stand gives you feedback: they take their role in supporting new acts seriously and give you a review if you want one. I wrote to ask for comments the next day and the reply said my performance and material had merits. They offered me another five minutes in December, which I accepted.

So, for December's set, I felt sufficiently emboldened to produce something new, to push myself to work further at these therapy/stand-up connections I am interested in and to work at them with this broader audience in mind.

I wrote. As the day approached I rehearsed under my breath, as before, as I walked up the hill to work. I dug out the hairbrush mic and I stood in our back room, regaling the walls, shrubs and trees of the courtyards beyond the window.

I was less rigorous, though. I felt confident. I did not time my set in my rehearsals. On the evidence of July, my thinking went, I clearly had more time than I felt I had. I knew the techie would flash a green light at me a minute or so before my time was up, and again when I have to get off stage, so I told myself I would know and be able to finish wherever it is I had got to.

I rehearsed again on the train back from Carlisle that afternoon, muttering my lines to a full carriage. The day before, a Sunday, I had done a dry run to Tess as we travelled home from a bright winter beach walk. She had laughed. I felt encouraged.

The green room, a tight, airless squeeze of space with old sofas and dirty carpets—and no green in sight—is busy at Red Raw. Ten acts. No Frankie Boyle this time. Some of us, the least experienced performers like me, get the five minutes and the more experienced get ten, with a mix of each of these alternating either side of the first interval. After a second interval the headliner, who might be well known, at least in Edinburgh or Scotland, does twenty minutes to finish the night's entertainment. The show is, as usual, held together by an MC, on this occasion a raucous, irrepressible young Scottish woman who, the audience realized early, took no prisoners.

I was on early, second, after the MC had warmed up the audience and following the first act, a man from London I remember enjoying but whose content I remember nothing about. I stood waiting at the threshold between four doors, the doors to the green room, the toilet, outside and the club itself. The MC returned to the stage as he ended, leading the applause for him, and then called on the audience to summon me with whooping and clapping.

***

I pass through the threshold door into the tight crowd. The MC and I pass and shake hands, and I'm there and it's familiar and comfortable. It feels good to be on the small, semi-circular, wooden platform. My gallows.

Detach mic, lift the stand out of the way, and begin.

The comedy rule is you must get a laugh within the first seconds. Find a quick line that'll break the ice and let them know you're ok. If you're ok, they're ok. On the other hand, if you open with, say, a statement like, "You need to know everything that happens from now is material for a book I'm writing", anyone will tell you it's not likely to go well. Instead, you sound smug and manipulative and someone not to trust. If you then move on to complain to the audience about only being given five minutes, if you also distance yourself from the usual comedy fare of jokes about failed sex, which *you're* not going to do, the declaring of all of which you have imagined will captivate the audience with its hilarious and obvious ironic self-deprecation, the crack in the floor will begin to open to the chasm below.

In this moment, if you're alert, what you should do is 'fess up, because, after all, as you've said in a previous set, in stand-up you have to make judgements in the moment, in the thick of it. You should make explicit to your still-willing audience you can see what's happening, you should be open with them that you've got off on the wrong foot, and offer a reflexive insight that reassures them you're experienced enough to work with the immediacy of the here-and-now dynamics. You might say, something like, "this isn't going so well, is it? Perhaps I'll just leave now", and pretend to walk off the stage. The audience will laugh and you're back on track.

That's not what happens. Instead, I plough my relentless furrow. I tell my poor, captive audience how doing stand-up is therapy for me these days and, boy, do I need it because I have no friends, my son has emigrated to the USA, and I'm ageing and losing hope. Note I deliver this when everyone present already sees me as obnoxious and can therefore quite believe I am both miserable and friendless, and deserve to be.[298]

Now, even now, there's a way to handle this. You cut your losses and leave the stage. You check your watch, see your time is not far off being up, and you leave the stage. You're polite, you're self-deprecating, you say, "Thank you for bearing with me. I'll be off then. I'm heading back to my drawing-board".

That's not what happens. I stay. I have more, much more. I haven't rehearsed the timing and I keep going and going and going, and the green light—that well-known signal every performer needs to respect—flashes to warns me I have a minute left to wrap up. I don't notice it. Jenny, the techie, flashes the green light again a minute later. I still don't see it. When 'Reet Petite' blasts from the sound system I stand for one, two, three, four seconds, too long, unable to register what's taking place. Leave, Jonathan, I should say to myself, get off, go, please go. At last, I get it, and I fumble the mic back into the stand and, to relieved applause, leave, passing the MC on the way. She shakes my hand and tries to smile.

In the green room, no one looks. Conversations continue. It's like I am marked, stained. It's like I am carrying the presence of death. Ignored, I do not exist. I don't blame them. What can they say?

When the interval comes, I gather my coat and leave.

Next day, imagining what to expect, I email to ask for feedback. The administrator replies to me. Jenny the technician had comments for me.

"Hi Jonathan,
Yes what you did wasn't stand-up so that's why it didn't go well. Feedback from Jenny below for you.
Best, Ellen
Jonathan Wyatt—Literally no jokes. Not one. And no stories either. He started by explaining that he's a therapist which explained why

his set felt like some weird social experiment. He then pretty much slagged comedians and weegies[299] alike by listing things he imagines the audience want (e.g. 'I imagine you want something more than just failed sex stories and profanities') but what he proceeded to do was NOT give the audience anything he imagined they wanted. He got one (and I really mean ONE) titter, about 1.5mins in, when he said, 'Therapists are supposed to get therapy too . . . it's a pyramid scheme'and that was it—the only thing slightly resembling something that might just be mildly amusing. I flashed him more than I've ever flashed anyone. Constant flashing when he hit 6 mins and then I cut him off. This just wasn't comedy".

* * *

I stop and lift up my head from the screen, reaching my arms up and out, rolling my shoulders. Shame isn't good for your posture. There are naval ships passing up river, from right to left, towards the Faslane nuclear base. They seem not to be in a rush, each in turn passing out of sight behind the cherry tree for some seconds. I stand, pick up the binoculars, thinking I will take a closer look but I find I am distracted by a black cat[300] stalking at the end of the garden. Through the glasses I follow her lithe determination to catch its prey.

Both Rafa's story and mine are both perhaps stories of abjection, "something rejected from which one is not separated".[301] For Limon, all stand-up is about abjection, and all stand-up a theory of what to do with it:

> All stand ups are abject in so far as they give themselves over to the stand-up condition, which is a non-condition between nature and artifice. (They are neither acting nor conversing, neither in nor out of costume). Reality itself, in the way of the abject, keeps returning to the stand-up comedian, who throws it off in the form of jokes. Obliviousness is earned from moment to moment.[302]

"It's only stand-up. Hold onto that", was my exhortation early in this section of the chapter. It's only stand-up, as if stand-up is not also real.[303] It is that "non-condition", that threshold, between "nature (sic) and artifice". If it were only artifice we wouldn't care. We remain attached to the abject. If we don't, if it were only sham, there would be no shame.[304] My shame arose from and through my inability to "throw off" my continuing abjection; and my cruelty, if that's what it was, came from placing Rafa in a position where there was no place in the story for him to throw off his. In my December Red Raw set, there was some truth in what I told the audience about being unhappy and lonely—there needed to be—but I did not, could not, convey how I was also at ease with that and how light, how *funny*, it also was. With Rafa, the shame stayed with him. I left his shame there, locking it to him as I threw him and his shame off and away from all those of us in that basement, with a dismissive "it's time you got your shit together".

It would have been different had Rafa had the last word:

Counselling: Stand-Up on Legs (alternative ending)

So, I'm here, in the moment, this broken, regretful young man and me in a dull-lit room in a non-descript building in a quiet Edinburgh suburb on an early Tuesday evening, and I look to stand-up for help: I become alert to timing, to notions of truth, to vulnerability, and I say, "Rafa, I can see that this has been an awful time for you. But—and I want you to look at me here—"

He does look at me. He stares. The shame is still there in his eyes, in the way he holds himself, but there's also determination, a rage even, that surprises me. He interrupts, taking the opportunity offered by my punchline-seeking pause:

"Yes, I know what's coming. I saw it a long way off. We all did."

He stands, picks up his coat, and walks to the door: "If you're going to pursue this stand-up career of yours, you need to—how shall I put it?—get your shit together".

I've been Jonathan Wyatt, counsellor. Thanks for listening.

***

May 2017. I am still in Kilcreggan. There's a trace of dissatisfaction, as I write, with where I have reached. It's been arduous to write this and I'm trying to work further into why. The writing clouds seem to have sunk low over me, like those I can see descending over the Clyde. The estuary waters seem stilled from this distance, their gray-green surface tranquilized, the pause button pressed on their relentless movement. The naval ships have long gone. The black cat too. The trees leading down from the house to the water's edge appear stiff, the mild wind causing leaves on exposed branches to sway but only barely.

The landscape craves a storm to disturb it, to shake it all up, to clear the air so we can see the mountains of Arran again, as we could on our first evening when at our horizon their peaks and edges cut the sky.

Where is the Cailleach, the Celtic goddess of storms and the one who made those mountains, when you need her? When you need her hibernal rage to return, just for a time, and keep Spring at bay?[305] These stories I have told risk rendering us all becalmed: Rafa, me, the audiences, Sarah. You. With no room to manoeuvre, no space to breathe.

Blow, Cailleach, blow. Blow this discourse, this talk of Rafa and me, shame, Sarah, my 'cruelty' or otherwise, my stand-up 'death', into something strange. Something that will loosen us, this. Something creative-relational.

Blow, Cailleach, blow.

Here might be the dissatisfaction I am in touch with: it is how the stories suggest a discourse of fixity, a discourse of the humanist personal, a transcendent ontology that positions me as outside Rafa, and Rafa as the 'other', over there; the audiences, if we think of the term, 'audience', etymologically, as passive, as 'those who hear' and only hear; Sarah, as disconnected, outside these various encounters, watching on a screen from afar in her kitchen at home; you, as a reader, now, as where you are, and only there; all of us at these various degrees of ontological separation. The stories, and my commentary on them, risk, too, casting shame as 'individual'. Mine, Rafa's.

Blow, Cailleach, blow.

I can't know where she would take us, where her winds would land us, and it may be towards a harsher, more troubling, assemblage, but I know it would not be this stasis. Different questions, disruptions, incitements.

Blow, Cailleach, blow.

Blow, Cailleach, blow.

***

She hears, she thunders:

What if we follow, she asks, not bodies (human or otherwise), but affect? What if we follow affect in the sense that Manning proposes, the "complex affective process[es] that . . . retain the collectivity at the heart of its having come-to-be"?[306] Affect that "activates the threshold that disperses it"? And what if we follow shame not as interior, not as 'owned' by any one human body but as an "affect that crosses many different orders of bodies"?[307] In other words not, for example, what is the 'unsayable' that should not have been said, nor what actions 'I' should have taken to rescue my set, but what thresholds did these events activate? What did they take me, us, towards?

Barad speaks of the problems with the feminist 'critique' of science, declaring uneasiness at how critique essentializes, how it closes down rather than opens up to what is to come. When the Cailleach blows across the Clyde estuary to Arran, when she howls into my rendering of the stories of both Rafa and me and The Stand, she disrupts, folding and rolling the water into land, land into water, stage into audience, therapy into stand-up into writing, Rafa into Sarah into me into the beers held in clenched fingers, the raging power of the storm goddess forging what Barad calls, *trans/materialities*, which "signal material intra-relatings and differences across, among, and between genders, species, spaces, knowledges, sexualities, subjectivities, and temporalities".[308]

The point is not that this lets anyone off the hook. The *trans/material* landscape of my comedy club stories and their aftermath after the Cailleach has made her mark leaves all its actors implicated. The newly disturbed, re-distributed, re-conceptualized intra-relatings speak instead of a mutual indebtedness in our own co-creation.

After the Cailleach has passed, an immanent, diffractive reading rather than a reading of critique feels possible, one that opens up, cutting together/apart, one move,[309] enabling us to become in touch with the work of 'worlding', "[the] sensory refrain pulling in events and scenes as if they were much-needed raw materials for a compositional grounding, a restart".[310] Such a "restart" is challenging to identify as it surfaces but it might be something like this. Hear, picture, sense what follows as hyphenated.

Rafa in the consulting room with me, the Rafa in and of my imagination, the two of us, him-and-me, with the audience and with Sarah; the 'me' of and in those five-minutes-that-became-six. Hear, see—sense— all of us on stage and all of us in the front row and all of us at the back, the lights illuminating the stage with the rest of that basement dulled, heeding or not the green-lit summons; and all of us—stage and lights and dark and human and other bodies—wondering: What-now?

Where-are-we-left? What-might-be-possible? How-has-this-come-to-be? What-are-the-forces-at-work-here? What-is-together-shit-anyway?

Blow, Cailleach, blow. "Blow, winds, and crack your cheeks".[311]

Some paragraphs back, I wondered if the question once the Cailleach had done her unruly work might be not what is the 'unsayable' that should not have been said, not what rescuing actions I should have taken, but *what thresholds do these events take me, us, towards*? I asked this at the time as a provocation, to help shift the stuck place it felt this engagement with shame, therapy and stand-up had reached. It was a question I thought I could leave open and intriguing, hanging unanswered, as if we could ever get close to it.

What thresholds do these events take me, us, towards? What is the restart the Cailleach has offered?

It is a troubling question, because thresholds are suggestive of uncertainty; they hint at the uneasy as well as the possible.

Like, how, as I look up the estuary waters and the trees begin to sway, I see the sadness in Rafa but also, the edges of his defiance and ire, the force, the possible, that he is; and the possible that therapy is.

Like, how, if stand-up concerns the constant 'throwing off' of abjection, as Limon suggests, how can that be sustainable? At what cost? And what else might be possible? What might be a way of doing stand-up otherwise?

NOTES

284 'Bright Club', as a reminder, is an evening of 'academic' stand-up; researchers doing stand-up about their research. See Chapters 6 and 7.

285 There is a film of a performance of this set here: www.youtube.com/watch?v=0skNeJB7eqY&t=43s

286 See Chapter 7.

287 I do not believe myself here. I would challenge, or would wish, to nuance this claim. Both stand-up and therapy are about more than helping us 'feel better', whatever that might mean. But the claim served my purpose.

288 Again, I would want to trouble this claim. Stewart Lee, in his 2016 show, "Content Provider", calls out this attribution to stand-up, stating in mock exasperation how if something was unsayable the performer wouldn't be saying it.

289 This too is contestable. Stand-up gives the appearance of spontaneity but for most performers it is scripted and rehearsed.

290 Within months of writing this set it was out of date. In the UK there is less need to draw cash now.

291 As I became more confident, I would make 'look into my eyes' gestures with one hand and lengthen the pause.

292 For support for this view see, for example, Bollas, *Forces of Destiny*, 1989; Lemma, *Humour on the Couch*, 2000; and Shearer, *Why Don't Psychotherapists Laugh*, 2016. Nick Barwick writes about the value and importance of humour in handling our developmental experiences of humiliation and shame. Barwick, "Looking on the Bright Side", 2012.

293 I think of this as working with and learning from the 'countertransference', i.e. that which is being experienced by the therapist. There is an extensive psychodynamic literature on this. Casement, *On Learning from the Patient*, 1985 is one source on understanding and working with the countertransference. I keep returning to him.

294 Berlant and Ngai, "Comedy Has Issues", 2017, 242.

295 Probyn, "Writing Shame", 2010.

296 Probyn, 74.

297 See Chapter 7.

298 Including my fellow performers behind me in the green room who, I imagine, were staring in disbelief at the green room's audio speaker as it channelled this unfolding disaster.

299 People from Glasgow. I was not aware I had done this. I did not feel open enough to further feedback to ask for clarification.

300 Unrelated, I assume, to the tabby of Chapter 5.

301 Kristeva, "Approaching Abjection", 1982, 127.

302 Limon, *Stand-up Comedy in Theory*, 2000, 105.

303 See page 141 for a brief discussion of 'real'.

304 Probyn, "Writing Shame", 2010.

305 For further information on the Cailleach, see Monaghan, Patricia, *The Encyclopedia of Celtic Mythology and Folklore*. New York: Facts on File, 2014; and Chapter 7, "Saving the Forest", in Galbraith, Alison and Alette Willis, *Dancing with Trees: Eco-Tales from the British Isles*. Stroud: The History Press, 2017.

306 Manning, *Always More Than One*, 2013, 28.

307 Probyn, "Writing Shame", 2010, 82.

308 Juelskjær and Schwennesn, "Intra-active Entanglements", 2012, 16.

309 Barad, "Diffracting Diffraction", 2014.

310 Stewart, *Ordinary Affects*, 2010, 350.

311 Shakespeare, *King Lear*, 3.2.1, 2013.

CHAPTER 13

MEDITATION ON A GREEN LIGHT BULB[312]

March-April 2018, Edinburgh

This chapter is a meditation on being given the green light and not taking it. A meditation on permission, a meditation on warning: on the insistent green flash the performer heeds or ignores; and the invitations the client gives—there, then gone—there, then gone—there, then gone—that the therapist might miss but sometimes take. It is a meditation on shame, regret and also hope.

1

Green Light Bulb

Green is go
Green is a call, a summons, a prompt

A light bulb
is straight and
curving glass

Green is raw
Green is young,
Green is growing
Green is naive

A light bulb
is incandescent with tungsten filament
and conductors

Green is life
Green is nature, safety, soothing

A light bulb
is a silent vacuum
empty, replete with absence

Green is life
Green is nature, raging, troubled
Green is life
Green is nature, this room, this floor

A light bulb
is a teeming vacuum
"the scene of wild activities"[313]

Green is open
Green is inviting, ready, accepting

A light bulb
is a hedonist vacuum,
a "jubilant exploration of virtuality"[314]

Green is open,
Green is welcome, inclusive, available

A light bulb
is a debauched absence
full of "virtual particles . . . having a field day"[315]

Green is envy
Green is reaching, yearning, loss

A light bulb
is incandescent with noble gas
with xenon, or krypton or helium, or mercury vapour or neon, or
argon

Green is envy
Green is destructive, violent, loss

A light bulb, incandescent with argon,
charged, coursing with fire through phosphors
becomes alive as green

Green is go
Green is permission, invitation, welcome

> A light bulb,
>   coursing with fire in argon through phosphors,
>   is incandescent with go, leave, go

Green is go
Green is go, leave, go

2

Waiting

> Waiting

> The stage is set: empty, open,
> hugged by tables and chairs that spread
> like dead leaves on autumn ground
> meeting blood-red walls

> Waiting

> The stage is set: the quiet mic on its stand,
> metal bodies resting on wooden floor-body
> human bodies pour in and pour themselves
> onto chairs and liquid bodies down open throats

> Waiting

> The stage is set: the mic on its stand shudders
> with its own expectancy, touching itself—
> "touched by all possible others"[316]
> all others, there and not there, then and not then

> Waiting

> The MC struts and swears, mic in hand,
> soft shoes, sharp eyes, keen tongue

the first laughters, then again, then again
rolling the room into the night, heat rising

Waiting

She calls, she shouts, she rouses, she summons
the man onto that stage. He's quiet, he's slow
quiet feels its way, a hush, a pause, a puzzle
a doubt, the mic heavy in his hand

Not waiting, now

A light show only for him, an explosion in his eye
there, gone, there, gone, there, gone,
an explosion he does not see, will not see
and subtle light gives way to brutal sound

3

7 Questions to the Green Light Bulb

1. Did you know what was happening?
2. What does it mean for you to know or not know?
3. Did you care?
4. What does it mean for you to care or not care?
5. Were you, do you think, morally neutral?
6. Is such a stance possible?
7. Are you familiar with shame?

4

Therapy Signals: With Karl

when the moment arises
as if from nowhere
a moment you're not searching for
a moment that takes you by surprise

a moment you know will come, sometime
now you sense it, now you don't

in the 'minor gestures'[317] of eyes lifting
or when he says nothing
but his sigh reaches out
against the pale wall and
brushes your cheek
now you sense it, now you don't

or a gust of wind outside
lifts then eases the leaves,
a glimpse in the corner of your eye,
or a cat passes the window
its soft, tabby fur flattening
now you sense it, now you don't

or when he reaches for water
like he does, like he always does
only this time there's a catch in the move
a signal, a flash, a clustering,
an opening, an invitation, a call
which now you sense, and now you don't

Notes

312 I presented a version of this chapter at the International Congress of Qualitative Inquiry, 2018, as part of a panel on "Ordinary Objects", curated by Stacy Holman Jones.

313 Cao and Schweber, 1993, 39.

314 Barad, "On Touching", 2012, 210.

315 Barad, 210.

316 Barad, 212.

317 Manning, *The Minor Gesture*, 2016.

CHAPTER 14

A THIRD STORY OF SHAME

Hannah Gadsby

Summer 2017 and July 2018, Edinburgh and Bristol

In this third story of shame I engage with Hannah Gadsby's show, Nanette, which I witnessed at the August 2017 Fringe. The performance is about how she is giving up comedy, both a show and a decision in which shame is significant. At the end of the chapter I return to both Elspeth Probyn and the Cailleach.

It's August again. 2017. The Fringe. An evening in another over-heated basement classroom-turned-theatre.[318] Outside it's cold and damp again. It's cramped again: the seats are fixed in rows, five or six deep, each with a fixed 'ledge', extended across the row, for taking notes or doodling in lectures. We are in the second row back (the resistance to sitting in the front row was successful this time, despite the prospect of greater leg room), towards the centre. There is barely enough room between us to shift position. Students must have got smaller over the years or, more likely, the university in its neo-liberal ambition must, like airlines, be shrinking its lecture theatre seat sizes in order to cram in more 'customers'.

Early in *Nanette*,[319] her hour-long show, Hannah Gadsby tells us she is finishing with stand-up, that she can't do it any longer. She is also in pain this evening, with wisdom tooth trouble. On a stool next to her there's an ice-pop that she picks up, wincing, to hold to her cheek every few minutes. Halfway through the set, one of the runners hovers at the side, replacement ice-pop ready on a shiny steel tray. He brings it in only when Gadsby summons him.

Gadsby is quitting stand-up after ten years. It's not because she's not successful. She's good at this game, she tells us. She's "a funny fucker". No, the problem with comedy, she says, is the required and, she implies, formulaic, restrictive incompleteness, the requirement to leave us with laughter, the metre of set-up and punchline, set-up, punchline, set-up, punchline. The "you gotta laugh" imperative. Her job—and therefore our expectation of her—is to create tension and then for her to release it with humour. Tension, release. Tension, release. Tension, release. How, she wonders, do people argue that comedy is good for us, therapeutic? Anxiety is introduced in us that was not there before, tension we did not enter the room with. And the requirement to release it, and mostly at her own expense—for her to be a funny fucker—means too much has to be left out. She can't keep doing it, she says. It's costing her too much.

Gadsby is known as a lesbian comic ("my people, the Lesbecians . . ."). She gives us the story of how, in a previous show, an audience member, "one of my people", approached her after a gig ("when of course I am going to be so open to feedback") to tell Gadsby how disappointed she had been, as had been others. "Even your own people are disappointed", the generous provider of helpful criticism told her: "there wasn't enough lesbian content" in the show. Gadsby points to her body and tells us, "But I was there all the time. Lesbian content".

Her show is never light but she is gentle on us for the first half-hour, explaining the origins of the show's title, which is the name of the barista in a small town in Australia she visited at the time when the pressure was on for her to produce a title. Nanette sounded to her like it would be the name of someone warm, nurturing and friendly. Nanette: a small nana (grandmother), and she loves nanas, so that's the title she landed on; the name of her surely grandmotherly barista. But her small-town barista was not surely but surly, suspicious and unwilling, which takes Gadsby— via a diatribe on Picasso's misogyny and the representation of women in renaissance art (she studied art history)—into a segment about the small town in northwestern Tasmania where she was brought up and about the reason she is giving up stand-up.

Her early stand-up shows were about growing up with her parents and brothers and coming out in this small town: the loneliness, the religious bigotry, the embarrassing, humiliating moments, like when the young teenage Gadsby, afraid of heights and uneasy with her growing and (to her) over-sized body, took the child's slide on a visit to the water park and became wedged on one sharp turn. We laugh with her at the image of the build-up of water behind her, the stranding of the small boy ahead of her on the now-dried-up slide, and his horror at being engulfed by the ultimately released Gadsby and the mini-tsunami she had generated.

A staple story she would tell in her first show, which she retells to us, was how at seventeen she was waiting at a bus stop at the end of a night out. A guy threatened her because she—though he thought 'she' was a 'he'—was making eyes at his girlfriend. (Throughout the show Gadsby draws attention to her appearance, her body, her height, her size, her masculine 'set', making us laugh when she tells us of its advantages, "though nobody pays me more, surprisingly".) The guy approaching her at the bus stop pauses when his girlfriend corrects him and, puzzled, he turns and leaves her be. The story has always, she says, gone down well, and it gets a gentle laugh of relief and sympathy from us.

However, later in the set, she returns to the same story to say how stand-up has required her over the years to leave it unfinished for the sake of getting a laugh. She is tired of this. She can't do it anymore. She now can't not tell how it's true the guy began to walk away with his girlfriend—which is where the story as originally told ended—but what subsequently happened is he returned to punch to the ground and then kick the 17-year-old Gadsby, declaring if she was "one of those" then she had it coming anyway. Pause. Silence. "You gotta laugh", she says. That story needs telling, she declares, even if she is unable to—and shouldn't—relieve tension.

She also, for different reasons, can no longer keep telling the story she would always tell of her mother's response to Gadsby coming out to her in Gadsby's late teens. Her mother, hands in the kitchen sink, looks to the sky and implores, "Why are you telling me that? Why do I want to know?" (Her dad's response was, "Well, at least it wasn't one of the boys".) That story of her and her mother has gained sympathetic laughter and recognition too over the years, as it does now with us, but she tells us she and her mother have worked out their relationship and these days they are close and they understand each other. It is this ending of the story (or the story-so-far, at least) she has to leave out in stand-up because it elicits no laughs.

We need stories, she argues, we need a beginning, middle and an end, if there is one, and not only the mechanical requirement to ratchet up the pressure then release it.

The sharp levity of the first half of the set turns gradually to fury, a fury she has only recently discovered in herself. Her default position has always been to handle her shame by either sending herself up or having a nap. Not any longer. She would in the past read something on social media that angered her, switch off, shrug her shoulders and lie down. But last year, jet-lagged in a London hotel room, she read something about same-sex marriage that enraged her and she immediately posted a robust response that was shared widely and swiftly. Her post elicited an invitation to contribute an article on the subject to a leading US magazine. By the time the magazine had contacted her to issue the invitation, though, she had slept and no longer felt exercised.

However, on stage, holding an ice-pop to her cheek to soothe the immediate pain of her inflamed wisdom tooth, her anger screams from her body. All these years, she spits, of holding in her body the impact of relentless self-loathing, the abjection she would throw off by working audiences like us to a point where we laugh not only with her, but also at her;[320] all the experiences she has been unable to speak of, like the sexual abuse as a child, the rape by three men; the simple, quotidian experience of living in and with this unspeakable body: enough, enough, enough, she declares. This way of being has harmed her and no longer serves her; it does not lead to change.

There is no laughter in the squeezed lecture theatre. She does not lighten it for us, does not seek to protect us, does not make it easier. She calls men out, calls men to step up and take responsibility. She does not release the tension she has created. We sit, cramped, hot, uncomfortable. I look at my watch. I try to stretch out my legs but meet only the wooden back of the row of seats in front. I shift to lean forward, resting my hands on the table, but can stay there only a few moments and straighten up, then worry I am too tall for the people behind to see so slump forward again. If we had sat in the front row I would have been okay, I complain to myself. Why didn't we do that? There were seats free, and she is not one of those performers who pick on audiences. We would have been safe. We know that now.

The discomfort is not only physical. I want to stand but I can't. I want to leap up and move. It, she, is riveting. I don't want her to stop; and, at the same time, I want to leave. I am being thrown around, buffeted by the energies she is unleashing. Gadsby is the Cailleach, the storm goddess, sweating and spitting under the lights as she gives vent to her anger; and to be here it is extraordinary and uneasy.

I want to leave, I realize, not only to relieve the tension, but also to act. To do stand-up again and do it differently. It would not, could not, be stand-up that moves me this way, stand-up that catches me up in its force, that swirls, that hurls us around like the Cailleach did in the house above the Clyde estuary, but it would be, could be, stand-up performed as if it were the last time.

The show finishes. She leaves the stage, the house lights come up, and the room empties fast. We climb the steps into the daylight and crowds around George Square and begin the twenty-minute walk home. I could dance all the way there and beyond.

***

The 23rd of July, 2018. The café where I am working at drawing this chapter to an end is by the harbourside in Bristol, in the southwest of England. I am here for a conference, which begins nearby along the water early this afternoon.

The harbourside has been 'regenerated' over recent years, complete with art galleries, restaurants, bars and cafés. Speaking of shame, on tourist websites there is little mention of the docks' history in Bristol's role as a leading slaving port.[321]

I have held back—writing has held back—from settling upon an ending to this short chapter. I have wondered whether it ends above with returning home from Hannah Gadsby, with that sense of having been galvanized by her show, by the potential for action in her writing/performing of shame. It does, I realize, but together also with this: how Gadsby's performance enacts, embodies, Probyn's description of the challenge of writing about shame:

> [S]hame is produced out of the clashing of mind and body, resulting in new acts of subjectivity consubstantial with the words in which they are expressed. Deleuze's idea of the subjective disposition allows us to understand something of the relationship between the writer, experience, expression, affect, and its effects. Shame cannot be conceived of as an external object that could be dispassionately described, nor is it a purely personal feeling. Shame is subjective in the strong sense of bringing into being an entity or an idea through the specific explosion of mind, body, place, and history.[322]

195

Hannah Gadsby's rendering of shame, neither as external object nor as (only) personal, was an explosion that brought into being a re-orienting, a reframing. Her writing/performance was an explosion of mind, body, place and history, like a visitation from the Cailleach, the Cailleach who can be called upon to re-cast what stand-up can do, what writing can do—and, perhaps, what therapy can do—and do otherwise.

NOTES

318 See Chapter 3.

319 The show is now on Netflix and has been widely lauded. www.theguardian.com/stage/2017/aug/19/hannah-gadsby-review-nanette

320 Limon, *Stand-up Comedy in Theory*, 2000.

321 See, for example: "Visit Bristol", https://visitbristol.co.uk/about-bristol/areas/harbourside

322 Probyn, "Writing Shame", 2010, 81.

EPILOGUE

Although an epilogue has the familiar meaning of being an 'ending', it is not necessarily so. 'Epilogue' carries the etymological meaning, 'words that are attached' ('epi-logos'). It is also therefore possible to see an epilogue as offering an always-present excess: as being still in the middle. There are no endings (or beginnings), only flows.[323]

July 2018, Edinburgh

Therapy: Karl

Karl takes his fork and stabs his chips. He eats two, then a half-hearted third, but he's not sure. Not sure he's interested any more. When Shell comes back she mutters something under her breath as she sits back down.

"What's that?"

"You weren't meant to hear. Nothing".

"Go on. Say".

"Your chip-chasing habit".

"Ah, right".

"I wouldn't miss that".

"No". He noticed the 'wouldn't'. She could have said 'won't'. He notices an unfamiliar lurch of hope.

He leaves the remaining chips in peace and places his knife and fork together.

She leans forward. "I'll bet you don't take that to him".

"No", he agrees. "They've not been uppermost in our discourse. My eating habits".

"Oo, get you. 'Discourse'". A swipe he expected—and deserves, he knows—but there's a playfulness in her tone he hasn't heard for months.

"Thank you", he bows. "Though I'm not sure how much longer we'll be continuing".

She looks at him. She looks at his face and not the forlorn chips. "What do you mean?"

"I think it might be time to stop. Well, nearly. I don't know, but I think so. I don't know how much more I have to say, or we have to say. Or do. Not sure there's more to be gained. Given, you know, things. Us. This".

"What does he say about it? Has he mentioned finishing?"

"No, not in so many words. He hasn't said, you know, "Enough, Karl. Begone. We're done here". We talk about it every so often, keep an eye on how it's going. I know there are time limits. But it's up to me too. Up to him and me".

She picks up her jacket as she sits.

"I think I'll talk about it with him next time", he declares.

"Well, do then", she says. He hears a mild impatience, which he understands. After all, it's not up to her. What can she say?

He pushes his plate away. "Okay. Let's go".

They pay the bill, which they split, and leave. She holds the door open for him as they step outside into the evening warmth. A heat has settled on the city this summer, sustained not just for the usual Edinburgh summer few minutes, or a lucky few hours, before clouds and rain spoil the fun, but for weeks. They walk beside each other, not touching, taking their route home across The Meadows. Clusters of young people are gathered on the grass. Some throw slick, or less than slick, frisbee passes to each other. Most sit, cupping beer cans or leaning back on tanned arms around improvised barbecues that release smoke upwards, undisturbed.

"What's it done for you, this therapy?", she asks as they stroll.

He doesn't answer for a few steps.

"I know that's a hard question", she adds. "A non-question, even".

They walk a few more paces. "I can't say", he says. "Not yet. But it's given me this, at least".

"Given you what?"

"A little more time".

She picks up a wayward frisbee that has slid to her feet and flicks it back whence it came.

He stops walking to watch the young woman near them catch it and throw it on. "And", he turns to her, "I feel . . . I feel I can move".

"That's good, that's good", she says.

Further on, a few paces before the crossing at Melville Drive, he adds.

"But I know there's more to be done. I know that".

She turns to look at him. "Yes, I understand. Of course. There's always more".

Stand-Up: Return to Red Raw

It's 7.45pm. I walk up the hill and turn left onto Heriot Row. I am not hurrying, though I wonder about whether I will be too late to get a seat.

When I arrive at The Stand there is still a short queue up the steps to the road. It moves quickly. I pay my £3 (inflation bites). All the seats are taken so I go to my spot around the corner by the bar and perch there. Moments later they draw the curtain back to open up the seating area the far side of the stage and I head across to take a seat at the end of a row, two back from the green room door.

It's good, if uneasy, to be back. There is a row of friends in front of me. A guy with dark hair and sketchy beard approaches, greets them, talks for a while, says goodbye—"See yous later", in what I later learn is a Livingston accent—and walks through the green room door. He is performing. I am more envious than relieved.

The queue is too long for a beer. I wait and wait for it to diminish. It does, with about ten minutes to go. I get a 'Cowboy' lager, The Stand's own—Aha, I say to myself, I see what they did there—and return to my seat.[324] The lager is unpleasant.

Demelza, my Friday afternoon yoga teacher, arrives. She walks past me to a row two or three behind me to join others. I don't say hello. That would be too much like being a fan, which I am. She is a wonderful teacher: every class is different, she teaches us how to think-with-moving, how to conceptualize—"breathe in from your bones to your skin, breathe out and let the bones sink back"—and she makes us laugh, mostly with her own mistakes.

I close my eyes for a few moments and listen. Voices—no, 'voices' doesn't do it, because 'voices' sound owned, discrete and individual and the sound is more a pulp of pitches, tones, calls, cries and laughter that hover and dive, emerge and disappear, between the cracks of the musical soundtrack, The Slits' energetic, edgy version of *I Heard it Through the Grapevine*. "Losing you would mean my life would cease/Because you mean that much to me".[325] Joe gave me this track on one of the playlists he makes for birthdays, Father's Day and other celebrations.

'Soundtrack' is not right, I realize: The Slits are in the dynamic aural mix, along with other sounds, not lying passive in the background.

I open my eyes. The colours come into view: the rust-red pillars, the deep green and blue walls, the scattered posters pinned to most of the available spaces (a red and white Gary Little—*A Little Bit of Personal*, coming up in November—and Lucy Porter's blue and yellow *Consequences* in December). There are signs too, firm but amused, handwritten in white pen on the dark walls: "No phones, no filming, no recording (we take a hard line on that), no talking during the show (because it's rude)".

Two staff members patrol with benign smiles, collecting glasses. Both have ponytails and beards.

I am writing too fast. I worry I won't be able to read my notebook. I am overwhelmed by it all. Here, part of it, in it.

A young, twenties—most of this audience is young, twenties—woman and her boyfriend ask if the seats next to me are free, which they are. (We will not talk much as the evening goes on, except when they politely and apologetically wish to leave their seats in the intervals. I will tell them not to worry, each time. And then as the final act leaves the stage, the guy, having seen me writing through the breaks, will ask me if I am a journalist. I will tell him I am nearing the end of writing a book about the connections between therapy and stand-up; and as I finish my sentence I will see I have lost him but will be rescued by MC Sian, who returns to bid farewell.)

I could leave now, and this would be enough. I have expectation, excitement even, about the acts to follow, but the show itself might feel also a loss. When the first performer steps onto that wooden stage, into the white chalk circle, it will be a pull away, a drawing into awareness of my being part of an 'audience', a shift in energy in the room. Here, in this mo(ve)ment[326] now, is the white chalk circle: something is happening.

Writing: The Room at the Back

11.15am, Thursday, 26 July 2018.

My desk in the back room at home. The surprising quiet of courtyards and gardens, full and lush, beyond the open window with its upper sash drawn down. Most days I have written here this summer there have been children playing in the middle distance, or the persistent churning and whirring of unseen machinery. Today is almost silent. Just the occasional birdsong.

My laptop at the centre of the desk.

To the right, fresh coffee I have made, not quite strong enough.

An empty glass.

A set of keys.

Two piles of paperwork, one domestic, one writing-projects-in-waiting, both piles untouched for weeks.

To the left, two print-outs of the manuscript of earlier versions of this text, each in clear plastic sleeves, one from three months ago, read and annotated, the other from two weeks back, premature and neglected.

A guide to the Edinburgh Fringe, which begins next week. No shows yet booked.

An umbrella, which usually stays in my bag but has been redundant during these long, dry weeks of June and July.

On the desk's upper shelf, three stacks of books (including one Kindle). I have needed them there, to hand, for company.

A plastic pot of pens.

An unopened small green bottle of Korean liquor, Soju, a present from Joe when he returned from Seoul over two years ago. He advised I might not like it, and that it was strong, and I have not yet felt drawn.

On the wall behind, scattered photographs of family. In the centre of these, one of my mother, from two summers ago—or was it three?—holding her first great-grandchild, just a few days old. She is looking down at him, cradling him in the crook of her left arm, touching a foot, a tiny, blue-socked foot, with her right thumb and forefinger. It was a wedding, I remember, and Mum is looking bright in pink jacket and patterned shirt. Below that photo is one of the two of us, her and me, together at the same event, close-up, our heads touching, making faces to the camera, both of us laughing. I saw Mum on Sunday. I am glad I, we, still have her.

Beyond, beyond this room, this desk, the world turns. Much has changed since this book's beginning, back in Montjaux in 2014. Much has changed both personally and politically, both locally and globally. There has been an intensification of politics, and an amplified sense of uncertainty, risk and danger. The need for action is ever more pressing.

Producing this text, diffracting therapy, stand-up and writing towards, as and through creative-relational inquiry, has been a (minor) gesture[327] in that urgent work. It will, I hope, keep on becoming so, in the movement it activates and the encounters it prompts.

NOTES

323 Deleuze and Parnet, *Dialogues II*, 2002.

324 Remember the cowboy mural behind the performer. See page 12.

325 The Slits. *I Heard It through the Grapevine*. Composed by Norman Whitfield, and Barrett Strong. Produced by Rema. London: Island Records, 1979.

326 Davies and Gannon, *Doing Collective Biography*, 2006.

327 Manning, *The Minor Gesture*, 2016.

REFERENCES

Adams, Tony E. "Seeking Father: Relationally Reframing a T Troubled Love Story." *Qualitative Inquiry* 12, no. 4 (2006): 704–23.

Adams, Tony E., Stacy Holman Jones, and Carolyn Ellis. *Autoethnography: An Overview*. Oxford: Oxford University Press, 2014.

Aitchison, Claire, and Alison Lee. "Research Writing: Problems and Pedagogies." *Teaching in Higher Education* 11, no. 3 (2007): 265–78.

Allen, Tony. *Attitude: Wanna Make Something of It? The Secret of Stand-up Comedy*. Glastonbury: Gothic Image Publications, 2001.

Austin, John L. *How to Do Things with Words*. Oxford: Clarendon Press, 1962.

Badiou, Alain. *Ethics: An Essay on the Understanding of Evil*. Translated by Peter Hallward. London: Verso, 2002.

Banks, Iain. *The Crow Road*. London: Abacus, 1992.

Barad, Karen. "Posthumanist Performativity: Toward an Understanding of How Matter Comes to Matter." *Signs: Journal of Women in Culture and Society* 28, no. 3 (2003): 801–31.

Barad, Karen. *Meeting the Universe Halfway: Quantum Physics and the Entanglement of Matter and Meaning*. Durham & London: Duke University Press, 2007.

Barad, Karen. "Diffracting Diffraction: Cutting Together-Apart." *Parallax* 20, no. 3 (2014): 168–87.

Barwick, Nick. "Looking on the Bright Side of Life: Some Thoughts on Developmental and Defensive Uses of Humour." *Psychodynamic Practice* 18, no. 2 (2012): 163–79.

Bennett, Jane. *Vibrant Matter: A Political Ecology of Things*. Durham, NC: Duke University Press, 2010.

Berlant, Lauren, and Sianne Ngai. "Comedy Has Issues." *Critical Inquiry* 43, no. 2 (2017): 233–49.

Bertelsen, Lone, and Andrew Murphie. "An Ethics of Everyday Infinities and Powers: Felix Guattari on Affect and the Refrain." Chap. 6 In *The Affect Theory Reader*, edited by Melissa Gregg and Gregory J. Seigworth, 138–57. Durham, NC: Duke University Press, 2010.

Biehl, João, and Peter Lock. "Deleuze and the Anthropology of Becoming." *Current Anthropology* 51, no. 3 (2010): 317–51.

Bochner, Arthur P, and Carolyn Ellis. "Communication as Autoethnography." In *Communication As . . . Perspectives on Theory*, edited by Gregory Shepherd, Jeffrey St. John and Ted Striphas, 110–22. Thousand Oaks: Sage, 2006.

Bogue, Ronald. *Deleuze on Music, Painting, and the Arts*. New York: Routledge, 2003.

Boldt, Gail, and Kevin Leander. "Becoming through 'the Break': A Post-Human Account of a Child's Play." *Journal of Early Childhood Literacy* 17, no. 3 (2017): 409–25.

Boldt, Gail, and Joseph M. Valente. "L'école Gulliver and La Borde: An Ethnographic Account of Collectivist Integration and Institutional Psychotherapy." *Curriculum Inquiry* 46, no. 3 (2016): 321–41. doi: https://doi.org/10.1080/03626784.2016.11 68260

Bollas, Christopher. *Forces of Destiny*. London: Free Association Press, 1989.

Borges, Jorge Luis. *Labyrinths*. Harmondsworth: Penguin, 1971.

Boutang, Pierre-André. *L'Abécédaire de Gilles Deleuze [Gilles Deleuze from A to Z]*. France: Semiotext(e), 1988.

Braidotti, Rosi. "Nomadism: Against Methodological Nationalism." *Policy Futures in Education* 8, no. 3–4 (2010): 408–18.

Braidotti, Rosi. *Nomadic Subjects*. New York: Columbia, 2011.

Brians, Ella. "The 'Virtual' Body and the Strange Persistence of the Flesh: Deleuze, Cyberspace and the Posthuman." Chap. 6 In *Deleuze and the Body*, edited by Laura Guillaume and Joe Hughes. Deleuze Connections, 117–43. Edinburgh: Edinburgh University Press, 2011.

Cao, Tian Yu, and Silvan S. Schweber. "The Conceptual Foundations and the Philosophical Aspects of Renormalization Theory." *Synthese* 97, no. 1 (1993): 33–108.

Casement, Patrick. *On Learning from the Patient*. London: Routledge, 2000.

Cavarero, Adriana. *Relating Narratives: Storytelling and Selfhood*. Translated by P.A. Kottman. London: Routledge, 2000.

Chun, Wendy Hui Kyong. *Updating to Remain the Same: Habitual Media*. Cambridge, MA: MIT Press, 2016.

Cixous, Hélène. "Coming to Writing." In *Coming to Writing and Other Essays*, edited by Deborah Jenson, 1–58. Cambridge, MA: Harvard University Press, 1991.

Cixous, Hélène. "Three Steps on the Ladder of Writing." In *The Hélène Cixous Reader*, edited by Susan Sellers, 199–205. London: Routledge, 1994.

Cixous, Hélène. *Stigmata*. London: Routledge, 2005, 1998.

Clough, Patrica Ticineto. *The User Unconscious: On Affect, Media and Measure*. Minneapolis: University of Minnesota, 2018.

Clough, Peter. *Narratives and Fictions in Educational Research*. Oxford: Oxford University Press, 2002.

Coles, Robert. *The Call of Stories*. Boston: Houghton Miflin, 1989.

Coole, Diana, and Samantha Frost, eds. *New Materialisms: Ontology, Agency, Politics*. Durham, NC: Duke University Press, 2010.

Cull, Laura. "Introduction." In *Deleuze and Performance*, edited by Laura Cull, 1–21. Edinburgh: Edinburgh University Press, 2009.

Davies, Bronwyn, and Susanne Gannon. *Doing Collective Biography: Investigating the Production of Subjectivity*. Buckingham: Open University Press, 2006.

Davies, Bronwyn, and Jonathan Wyatt. "Ethics." Chap. 4 In *Deleuze and Collaborative Writing: An Immanent Plane of Composition*, edited by Jonathan Wyatt, Ken Gale, Susanne Gannon and Bronwyn Davies, 105–29. New York: Peter Lang, 2011.

de Freitas, Elizabeth. "Karen Barad's Quantum Ontology and Posthuman Ethics: Rethinking the Concept of Relationality." *Qualitative Inquiry* 23, no. 9 (2017): 741–48.

Deleuze, Gilles. "Cours Vincennes 12/21/1980." www.webdeleuze.com/php/texte. php?cle=190andgroupe=Spinozaandlangue=2 (accessed 15 December 2017).

Deleuze, Gilles. *The Logic of Sense*. Translated by Mark Lester. New York: Columbia University Press, 1990.

Deleuze, Gilles. *Essays Critical and Clinical*. Translated by Daniel W. Smith and Michael A. Greco. London: Verso, 1998.

Deleuze, Gilles. *Difference and Repetition*. Translated by Paul Patton. London: Continuum, 2004.

Deleuze, Gilles, and Félix Guattari. *What Is Philosophy?* Translated by Hugh Tomlinson and Graham Burchell. New York: Columbia University Press, 1994.

Deleuze, Gilles, and Félix Guattari. *A Thousand Plateaus*. Translated by Brian Massumi. London: Continuum, 2004.

Deleuze, Gilles, and Claire Parnet. *Dialogues II*. Translated by Hugh Tomlinson. London: Continuum, 2002.

Derrida, Jacques. *The Work of Mourning*. Edited by P.-A. Braut and M. Naas. Chicago and London: The University of Chicago Press, 2003.

Dosse, Francois. *Gilles Deleuze & Felix Guattari: Intersecting Lives*. Translated by Deborah Glassman. Chichester, UK: Columbia, 2010.

Double, Oliver. *Getting the Joke: The Inner Workings of Stand-up Comedy*. London: Methuen, 2013.

Eliot, Thomas Stearns. *Four Quartets*. London: Faber & Faber, 2009.

Ellis, Carolyn. *The Ethnographic I: A Methodological Novel*. Walnut Creek, CA: Alta Mira, 2004.

Ellis, Carolyn. *Revision: Autoethnographic Reflections on Life and Work*. Walnut Creek, CA: Left Coast Press, 2009.

Ellis, Carolyn, Tony E. Adams, and Arthur P. Bochner. "Autoethnography: An Overview." *Historical Social Research/Historische Sozialforschung* (2011): 273–90.

Ellis, Carolyn, and Arthur P. Bochner. "Autoethnography, Personal Narrative, Reflexivity: Researcher as Subject." In *Handbook of Qualitative Research*, edited by N. K. and Y. S. Lincoln Denzin, 733–68. Thousand Oaks: Sage, 2000.

Ettinger, Bacha Lichtenberg. "From Transference to Aesthetic Paradigm: A Conversation with Felix Guattari." Chap. 15 In *A Shock to Thought: Expression after Deleuze and Guattari*, edited by Brian Massumi, 240–45. London: Routledge, 2002.

Fine, Michelle. "Working the Hyphens: Reinventing Self and Other in Qualitative Research." Chap. 4 In *Handbook of Qualitative Research*, edited by N. Denzin and Y. Lincoln, 70–82. Thousand Oaks, CA: Sage, 1994.

Ford, John. "The Man Who Shot Liberty Valance." 122 mins. Los Angeles: Paramount Pictures Corp, 1962.

Fritsch, Kelly. "Desiring Disability Differently: Neoliberalism, Heterotopic Imagination and Intra-Corporeal Reconfigurations." *Foucault Studies*, no. 19 (2015): 43–66.

Fulton, Alice. *Powers of Congress*. Louisville: Sarabande, 2001. 1990.

Gale, Ken. *Madness as Methodology: Bringing Concepts to Life in Contemporary Theorising and Inquiry*. London: Routledge, 2018.

Gale, Ken, Viv Martin, Artemi Sakellariadis, Jane Speedy, and Tami Spry. "Collaborative Writing in Real Time." *Qualitative Inquiry* 12, no. 5 (2012): 401–07.

Gale, Ken, Larry Russell, Ronald J. Pelias, Tami Spry, and Jonathan Wyatt. *How Writing Touches: An Intimate Scholarly Collaboration*. Newcastle-upon-Tyne: Cambridge Scholars Publishing, 2012.

Gale, Ken, and Jonathan Wyatt. "Writing the Incalculable: A Second Interactive Inquiry." *Qualitative Inquiry* 13, no. 6 (2007): 787–807.

Gale, Ken, and Jonathan Wyatt. *Between the Two: A Nomadic Inquiry into Collaborative Writing and Subjectivity*. Newcastle-upon-Tyne: Cambridge Scholars Publishing, 2009.

Gale, Ken, and Jonathan Wyatt. "Assemblage/Ethnography: Troubling Constructions of Self in the Play of Materiality and Representation." In *Contemporary British Autoethnography*, edited by Nigel Short, Lydia Turner and Alec Grant, 139–55. Rotterdam: Sense, 2013.

Gale, Ken, and Jonathan Wyatt. "Working at the Wonder: Collaborative Writing as Method of Inquiry." *Qualitative Inquiry* 23, no. 5 (2017): 355–64.

Gale, Ken, and Jonathan Wyatt. "Riding the Waves of Collaborative-Writing-as-Inquiry: Some Ontological Creative Detours." In *Cultivating Creativity in Methodology and Research: In Praise of Detours*, edited by Charlotte Wegener, Nina Meier and Eline Maslo, 193–205. London: Palgrave, 2018.

Gannon, Susanne. "Sketching Subjectivities." In *Handbook of Autoethnography*, edited by Tony E. Adams, Stacy Holman Jones and Carolyn Ellis, 228–43. Walnut Creek, CA: Left Coast Press, 2013.

Gilbert, Joanne R. *Performing Marginality: Humor, Gender, and Cultural Critique*. Detroit, MI: Wayne State University Press, 2004.

Goldstein, Kurt. *The Organism: A Holistic Approach to Biology Derived from Pathological Data in Man*. New York: American Book Company, 1939.

Gordon, Avery. *Ghostly Matters: Haunting and the Sociological Imagination*. London: University of Minnesota Press, 2008.

Guattari, Félix. *Chaosmosis*. Translated by Paul Bains and Julian Pefanis. Bloomington & Indianapolis, IN: Indiana University Press, 1995.

Guattari, Félix. *Chaosophy: Texts and Interviews 1972–77*. Translated by David L. Sweet, Jarred Becker and Taylor Adkins. Cambridge, MA: Semiotext(e), 2009.

Guattari, Félix. *Soft Subversions: Texts and Interviews 1977–1985*. Translated by Chet Wiener and Emily Wittman. Los Angeles, CA: Semiotext(e), 2009.

Harris, Anne. *The Creative Turn: Towards a New Aesthetic Imaginary*. Rotterdam: Sense, 2014.

Hemmingson, Michael. "Make Them Giggle: Auto/Ethnography as Stand-up Comedy." *Creative Approaches to Research* 1, no. 2 (2008): 9.

Huizinga, John. *Homo Ludens: A Study of the Play Element in Culture*. Abingdon, UK: Routledge, 2002, 10.

Hunter, Reginald D. *Reginald D. Hunter Live*. Orlando: Universal Studios, 2011.

Jackson, Alecia Youngblood. "An Ontology of a Backflip." *Cultural Studies <=> Critical Methodologies* 16, no. 2 (2016): 183–92.

Jackson, Alecia Youngblood. "Thinking without Method." *Qualitative Inquiry* 23, no. 9 (2017): 666–74.

Jackson, Alecia Youngblood, and Lisa A. Mazzei. "Experience and 'I' in Autoethnography: A Deconstruction." *International Review of Qualitative Research* 1, no. 3 (2008): 299–318.

Juelskjær, Malou, and Nete Schwennesn. "Intra-Active Entanglements—An Interview with Karen Barad." *Kvinder, køn & forskning*, no. 1–2 (2012): 10–23.

Krell, David F. *The Purest of Bastards: Works of Mourning, Art, and Affirmation in the Thought of Jacques Derrida*. University Park: Pennsylvania State University Press, 2000.

Kristeva, Julia. "Approaching Abjection." *Oxford Literary Review* 5, no. 1/2 (1982): 125–49.

Lee, Stewart. *How I Escaped My Certain Fate: The Life and Deaths of a Stand-up Comedian*. London: Faber, 2010.

Lemma, Alessandra. *Humour on the Couch*. London: Whurr, 2000.

Limon, John. *Stand-up Comedy in Theory, or, Abjection in America*. Durham, CA: Duke University Press, 2000.

MacDonald, Helen. *H Is for Hawk*. London: Jonathan Cape, 2014.

MacFarlane, Robert. *The Old Ways*. London: Penguin, 2012.

MacLure, Maggie. "The Refrain of the A-Grammatical Child: Finding Another Language in/for Qualitative Research." *Cultural Studie <=> Critical Methodologies* 16, no. 2 (2016): 173–82.

MacRury, Iain. "Humour as 'Social Dreaming': Stand-up Comedy as Therapeutic Performance." *Psychoanalysis, Culture & Society* 17, no. 2 (2012): 185–203.

Madison, D. Soyini. *Acts of Activism: Human Rights as Radical Performance*. New York: Cambridge University Press, 2010.

Manning, Erin. "Always More Than One: The Collectivity of *a Life*." *Body and Society* 16, no. 1 (2010): 117–27.

Manning, Erin. *Always More Than One: Individuation's Dance*. Minneapolis: University of Minnesota, 2013.

Manning, Erin, and Brian Massumi. *Thought in the Act: Passages in the Ecology of Experience*. Minneapolis: University of Minnesota, 2014.

Manning, Erin, and Brian Massumi. "Just Like That: William Forsythe: Between Movement and Language." In *Sentient Performativities of Embodiment*, edited by L. Hunter, E. Krimmer and P. Lichtenfels, 119–44. London: Lexington, 2016.

Massumi, Brian. "The Autonomy of Affect." *Cultural Critique*, no. 31 (1995): 83–109.

Massumi, Brian. "The Supernormal Animal." In *The Nonhuman Turn*, edited by Richard Grusin, 1–17. Minneapolis: University of Minnesota Press, 2015.

Mazzei, Lisa A. "Beyond an Easy Sense: A Diffractive Analysis." *Qualitative Inquiry* 20, no. 6 (2014): 742–46.

Mazzei, Lisa A., and Alecia Y. Jackson. *Thinking with Theory in Qualitative Research: Viewing Data across Multiple Perspectives*. London: Routledge, 2012.

McGregor, Jon. "My Working Day: 'I Have Never Been Asked How I Juggle Writing and Fatherhood. I'm Not Complaining'." *The Guardian*, 6 January 2018.

Murray, Fiona. "When Dust Gets in Your Eyes." *Capacious* 1, no. 1 (2017): 103–16.

Nancy, Jean-Luc. *Being Singular Plural*. Translated by Robert D. Richardson and Anne E. O'Byrne. Stanford: Stanford University Press, 2000.

Orlie, Melissa A. "Impersonal Matter." In *New Materialisms: Ontology, Agency and Politics*, edited by Diana Coole and Samantha Frost, 116–36. Durham, NC: Duke, 2010.

Pelias, Ronald J. *A Methodology of the Heart: Evoking Academic and Daily Life*. Oxford: AltaMira Press, 2004.

Pelias, Ronald J. "Performative Writing as Scholarship: An Apology, an Argument, an Anecdote." *Cultural Studies <=> Critical Methodologies* 5, no. 4 (2005): 415–24.

Pelias, Ronald J. "A Personal History of Lust on Bourbon Street." *Text and Performance Quarterly* 26, no. 1 (2006): 47–56.

Pelias, Ronald J. "Performative Writing Workshop." In *3rd International Congress of Qualitative Inquiry*. University of Illinois at Urbana-Champaign, 2007.

Pineau, Elyse. "Haunted by Ghosts: Collaborating with Absent Others." *International Review of Qualitative Research* 5, no. 4 (2012): 459–65.

Pollock, Della. "Performing Writing." In *The Ends of Performance*, edited by Peggy Phelan and Jill Lane, 73–103. London: New York University Press, 1998.

Poulos, Christopher N. "The Liminal Hero." *Cultural Studies <=> Critical Methodologies* 12, no. 6 (2012): 485–90.

Probyn, Elspeth. "Writing Shame." In *The Affect Theory Reader*, edited by Melissa Gregg and Gregory J. Seigworth, 71–90. Durham and London: Duke University Press, 2010.

Rajchman, John. *The Deleuze Connections*. London: The MIT Press, 2000.

Reed, Henry. *A Map of Verona*. London: Jonathan Cape, 1946.

Richardson, Laurel. "Writing: A Method of Inquiry." In *Handbook of Qualitative Research*, edited by Norman K. Denzin and Yvonna S. Lincoln, 516–29. London: Sage, 1994.

Richardson, Laurel. *Fields of Play (Constructing an Academic Life)*. New Brunswick: Rutgers University Press, 1997.

Richardson, Laurel. "Writing: A Method of Inquiry." In *Handbook of Qualitative Research*, edited by Norman Denzin and Yvonna Lincoln, 923–49. Thousand Oaks, CA: Sage, 2000.

Richardson, Laurel, and Elizabeth A. St Pierre. "Writing: A Method of Inquiry." In *Handbook of Qualitative Research*, edited by Norman K. Denzin and Yvonna S. Lincoln, 959–78. London: Sage, 2005.

Richardson, Laurel, and Elizabeth A. St. Piere. "Writing: A Method of Inquiry." Chap. 36 In *Handbook of Qualitative Research*, edited by Norman K. Denzin and Yvonna S. Lincoln, 818–38. London: Sage, 2017.

Rogers, Annie G., Mary E. Casey, Jennifer Ekert, James Holland, Victoria Nakkula, and Nurit Sheinburg. "An Interpretive Poetics of Languages of the Unsayable." In *Making Meaning of Narratives: The Narrative Study of Lives, Vol. 6*, edited by Ruthellen Josselson and Amia Lieblich, 77–106. London: Sage, 1999.

Saltmarsh, Sue. "Haunting Concepts in Social Research." *Discourse: Studies in the Cultural Politics of Education* 30, no. 4 (2009): 539–46.

Sedgwick, Eve Kosofsky. "A Dialogue on Love." *Critical Inquiry* 24, no. 2 (1998): 611–31.

Sellers, Susan, ed. *The Writing Notebooks of Hélène Cixous*. London: Continuum, 2004.

Shakespeare, William. *King Lear*, edited by Kenneth Muir. Arden Shakespeare, 9th edition. London: Methuen, 2013.

Shearer, Ann. *What Don't Psychotherapists Laugh? Enjoyment and the Consulting Room*. Abingdon: Routledge, 2016.

Short, Nigel, Lydia Turner, and Alec Grant, eds. *Contemporary British Autoethnography*. Rotterdam: Sense, 2013.

Siddique, Haroon. "Comedians Say Case of Sued Performer Is Threat to the Art." *The Guardian*, 23 February 2018.

Speedy, Jane. "Collaborative Writing and Ethical Know-How: Movements within the Space around Scholarship, the Academy and the Social Research Imaginary." *International Review of Qualitative Research* 5, no. 4 (2012): 349–56.

Speedy, Jane, Dave Bainton, Nell Bridges, Tony Brown, Laurinda Brown, Viv Martin, Artemi Sakellariadis, Susan Williams, and Sue Wilson. "Encountering 'Gerald': Experiments with Meandering Methodologies and Experiences Beyond Our 'Selves' in a Collaborative Writing Group." *Qualitative Inquiry* 16, no. 10 (2010): 894–901.

Springgay, Stephanie, and Sarah E. Truman. *Walking Methodologies in a More-Than-Human World: Walkinglab*. London: Routledge, 2018.

Spry, Tami. *Body, Paper, Stage: Writing and Performing Autoethnography*. Walnut Creek, CA: Left Coast Press, 2011.

St. Pierre, Elizabeth Adams. "Deleuzian Concepts for Education: The Subject Undone." *Educational Philosophy and Theory* 36, no. 3 (2004): 283–96.

St. Pierre, Elizabeth Adams. "Decentering Voice in Qualitative Inquiry." *International Review of Qualitative Research* 1, no. 3 (2008): 319–36.

St. Pierre, Elizabeth Adams. "Post Qualitative Research: The Critique and the Coming After." Chap. 37 In *The Sage Handbook of Qualitative Research*, edited by Norman K. Denzin and Yvonna S. Lincoln, 611–25. London: Sage, 2011.

St. Pierre, Elizabeth Adams. "The Posts Continue: Becoming." *International Journal of Qualitative Studies in Education* 26, no. 6 (2013): 646–57.

St. Pierre, Elizabeth Adams. "Deleuze and Guattari's Language for New Empirical Inquiry." *Educational Philosophy and Theory* 49, no. 11 (2017): 1080–89.

St. Pierre, Elizabeth A., Alecia Youngblood Jackson, and Lisa A. Mazzei. "New Empiricisms and New Materialisms: Conditions for New Inquiry." *Cultural Studie <=> Critical Methodologies* 16, no. 2 (2016): 99–110.

Stern, Daniel. *The Present Moment in Psychotherapy and Everyday Life*. New York: Norton, 2004.

Stevens, Wallace. *Harmonium*. London: Faber and Faber, 2001.

Stewart, Kathleen. *Ordinary Affects*. Durham, NC: Duke University Press, 2007.

Tamas, Sophie, and Jonathan Wyatt. "Telling." *Qualitative Inquiry* 19, no. 1 (2013): 60–66.

Turner, Lydia, Nigel Short, Alec Grant, and Tony E. Adams, eds. *International Perspectives on Autoethnographic Research and Practice*. London: Routledge, 2018.

Ulmer, Jasmin B. "Composing Techniques: Choreographing a Postqualitative Writing Practice." *Qualitative Inquiry*, no. 1-9 (2017).

Watson, Jannell. "Eco-Sensibilities: An Interview with Jane Bennett." *The Minnesota Review*, no. 81 (2013): 147-58.

White, Julie. *Permission: The International Interdisciplinary Impact of Laurel Richardson's Work*. Rotterdam: Sense, 2016.

White, Michael. *Reflections on Narrative Practice: Essays and Interviews*. Adelaide: Dulwich Centre Publications, 2000.

White, Michael. *Maps of Narrative Practice*. New York: Norton, 2007.

Wyatt, Jonathan. "A Gentle Going? An Autoethnographic Short Story." *Qualitative Inquiry* 11, no. 5 (2005): 724-32.

Wyatt, Jonathan. "Psychic Distance, Consent and Other Ethical Issues: Reflections on the Writing of 'a Gentle Going?'". *Qualitative Inquiry* 12, no. 4 (2006): 813-18.

Wyatt, Jonathan. "No Longer Loss: Autoethnographic Stammering." *Qualitative Inquiry* 14, no. 6 (2008): 955-67.

Wyatt, Jonathan. "What Kind of Mourning? Autoethnographic Fragments." *International Review of Qualitative Research* 2, no. 4 (2011): 499-512.

Wyatt, Jonathan. "Fathers, Sons, Loss and the Search for the Question." *Qualitative Inquiry* 18, no. 2 (2012): 162-67.

Wyatt, Jonathan. "Ash Wednesdays: An Autoethnography of (Not) Counselling." In *Contemporary British Autoethnography*, edited by Nigel Short, Lydia Turner and Alec Grant, 127-37. Rotterdam: Sense, 2013.

Wyatt, Jonathan. "Always in Thresholds." *Departures in Critical Qualitative Research* 3, no. 1 (2014): 8-17.

Wyatt, Jonathan, and Ken Gale. "Getting out of Selves: An Assemblage/Ethnography?" In *Handbook of Autoethnography*, edited by Tony E. Adams, Stacy Holman Jones and Carolyn Ellis, 300-12. Walnut Creek, CA: Left Coast, 2013.

Wyatt, Jonathan, and Ken Gale. "Writing to It: Creative Engagements with Writing Practice in and with the Not Yet Known in Today's Academy." *International Journal of Qualitative Studies in Education* 31, no. 2 (2018): 119-29.

Wyatt, Jonathan, Ken Gale, Larry Russell, Ronald J. Pelias, and Tami Spry. "How Writing Touches: An Intimate Scholarly Collaboration." *International Review of Qualitative Research* 4, no. 3 (2011): 253-77.

Wyatt, Jonathan, and Tess Wyatt. "(Be)Coming Home." In *Stories of Home: Place, Identity, Exile*, edited by Devika Chawla and Stacy Holman Jones, 31-46. Lanham, MD: Lexington, 2015.

INDEX

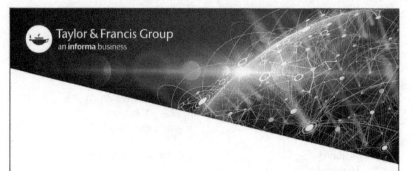